Clinical Nu
in the Community

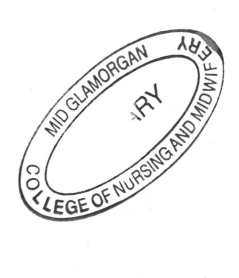

Other books of interest

The Royal Marsden Hospital Manual of Clinical Nursing Procedures
Third edition
Edited by P. Pritchard and J. Mallett
0–632–03387–8

Community Health Care Nursing
Edited by D. Sines
0–632–03856–X

Bolden & Takle's Practice Nurse Handbook
Third Edition
G. Hampson
0–632–03692–3

The Royal Marsden Hospital Manual of Standards of Care
Edited by J. Luthert and L. Robinson
0–632–03386–X

Health Visiting: Towards Community Health Nursing
Second Edition
Edited by K. Luker and J. Orr
0–632–03324–X

Care of People with Diabetes: A Manual of Nursing Practice
T. Dunning
0–632–03876–4

The Care of Wounds
C. Dealey
0–632–03864–0

Nursing in Nursing Homes
L. Nazarko
0–632–03987–6

Clinical Nursing Practice in the Community

Edited by

Maria Kenrick

Lecturer, Department of Nursing, University of Liverpool

and

Karen A. Luker

*Professor of Community Nursing, Department of Nursing,
University of Liverpool*

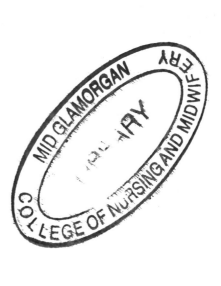

**Blackwell
Science**

© 1995 by
Blackwell Science Ltd
Editorial Offices:
Osney Mead, Oxford OX2 0EL
25 John Street, London WC1N 2BL
23 Ainslie Place, Edinburgh EH3 6AJ
238 Main Street, Cambridge
  Massachusetts 02142, USA
54 University Street, Carlton
  Victoria 3053, Australia

Other Editorial Offices:
Arnette Blackwell SA
1, rue de Lille, 75007 Paris
France

Blackwell Wissenschafts-Verlag GmbH
Kurfürstendamm 57
10707 Berlin, Germany

Blackwell MZV
Feldgasse 13, A-1238 Wien
Austria

First published 1995.

Set by DP Photosetting, Aylesbury, Bucks
Printed and bound in Great Britain by
The University Press, Cambridge.

DISTRIBUTORS

  Marston Book Services Ltd
  PO Box 87
  Oxford OX2 0DT
  (*Orders:* Tel: 01865 791155
         Fax: 01865 791927
         Telex: 837515)

North America
  Blackwell Science, Inc.
  238 Main Street
  Cambridge, MA 02142
  (*Orders:* Tel: 800 215-1000
         617 876-7000
         Fax: 617 492-5263)

Australia
  Blackwell Science Pty Ltd
  54 University Street
  Carlton, Victoria 3053
  (*Orders:* Tel: 03 347-5552)

A catalogue record for this title is available from
the British Library

ISBN 0–632–03858–6

Library of Congress
Cataloging-in-Publication Data is available.

Contents

Contributors

Maureen Benbow, *BA, RGN*, Tissue Viability Nurse, Mid Cheshire Hospitals Trust.

Ann-Louise Caress, *BNurs, RGN, RHV, NDNC*, Lecturer in Nursing, University of Liverpool.

Caroline Carlisle, *MSc, BA, RGN, RM, NDNC, Dip Counselling, RNT*, Lecturer in Nursing, University of Liverpool.

Nicky Cullum, *PhD, BSc(Hons), RGN*, Research Fellow, Centre for Health Economics, University of York.

Bernard Gibbon, *MSc, RGN, RMN, RNT*, Lecturer in Nursing, University of Liverpool.

Jane Griffiths, *BNurs(Hons), RGN, NDNC*, Queens Nursing Institute Research Associate.

Janet Hutchinson, *RGN, HV Cert, NDNC, MPH*, Public Health Adviser, Sefton Health.

Maria Kenrick, *RGN, BSc(Hons), MSc*, Lecturer in Nursing, University of Liverpool.

Karen A. Luker, *BNurs, PhD, RGN, RHV, NDNC*, Professor of Community Nursing, University of Liverpool.

E. Andrea Nelson, *BSc(Hons), RGN*, Lecturer in Nursing, University of Liverpool. Formerly; Research Associate, Lothian & Forth Valley Leg Ulcer Study.

Susan Noyce, *BPharm, MRPharmS*, Pharmaceutical Adviser, Sefton Health.

Ann Pursey, *PhD, BNurs(Hons), RGN, RHV*, Advanced Nursing Practitioner, Evesham Community Hospital.

Sonia E. Stott, *RGN, SCM, NDNC*, Senior Nurse, Continence Advisory Service, Central Manchester NHS Trust.

Susie M. Wilkinson, *PhD, RGN, MSc, RM, RCNT, RNT, ONC Cert, Cert Counselling, Dip Aromatherapy, Dip Nursing, Dip Ad Nursing Studies*, Director of Studies, Liverpool Marie Curie Centre.

Simon Woods, *RGN, ONC Cert, BA(Hons)*, Macmillan Lecturer in Cancer Nursing, University of Liverpool.

Introduction

Maria Kenrick and Karen A. Luker

COMMUNITY NURSING IN CONTEXT

The past decade has witnessed momentous political and organisational change in the National Health Service. Since the publication of the white paper *Working for Patients* (Department of Health, 1989a) there has been unprecedented change in the NHS and this change has particular significance for the primary health care field as most health care provision occurs in this sector. For the first time there is also a clear commitment from the government to move towards evidence based practice. Since April 1991 the NHS has had a research and development (R&D) strategy. The prime objective of this strategy is to ensure that:

> 'research and development becomes an integral part of health care, so that clinicians, managers and other staff find it natural to rely on the results of research in their day to day decision making and longer term strategic planning.'
> (Department of Health, 1991a, p1).

The centrality of R&D to the NHS is driven by the need to ensure that there is efficient and effective use of resources to improve the nation's health, and in this community nurses have their own part to play. The striving for consistently good practice has created a need for improved information about different treatments and forms of health care provision (Department of Health, 1992a). An excursion through the literature on community nursing makes one all too aware of how little is really known about our work. As the profession moves into the 21st century community nurses are having to adapt to radically different working practices and are increasingly being called upon to extend their skills and expand their clinical role. In order to provide a high quality of patient care it is now necessary that clinical decisions are based on available evidence. In some cases this means the findings of randomised controlled clinical trials whilst in others the evidence for practice is based on case histories or professional consensus. In this book we have drawn upon all these various authoritative sources when discussing practical procedures or other nursing interventions.

Since the reform of nursing education, commonly referred to as Project 2000 (United Kingdom Central Council for Nursing, Midwifery and Health Visiting, 1986) and the publication of the Strategy for Nursing (Department of Health 1989b) there have been four major policy initiatives which have had a considerable impact on the work of nurses in the community, namely:

- The NHS & Community Care Act 1990
- *The Patient's Charter* 1991
- *The Health of the Nation* (Department of Health, 1992b)
- The Strategy for Nursing, Midwifery and Health Visiting Research 1993.

The NHS and Community Care Act 1990

The 1990 NHS and Community Care Act has precipitated many changes in community nursing, as has the GP contract. There is now an imperative to provide a high quality and efficient service, often without the input of additional human or financial resources. This has resulted in diversification in the community nursing workforce and in some cases new roles and responsibilities have emerged.

The introduction of an internal market for care provision has brought the issue of 'Quality Care' to the top of the agenda (Department of Health, 1993). Purchasers and providers of health services are now obliged to incorporate quality control mechanisms into their contracting arrangements. Community nurses now have to demonstrate that they really do provide a high quality caring service to patients and their families. Community nurses, along with other health care professionals, are being required to subject their professional practices to the scrutiny of clinical audit, and to demonstrate in terms of measurable outcomes the utility of the services they provide.

With the advent of fund holding GPs, a great deal more secondary health care is now being provided in GP surgeries and patients' own homes, with a corresponding increase in demand for the services of community nurses. The general trend is towards earlier discharge from hospital, more patients having day case surgery and higher numbers of people with chronic and terminal illnesses being treated and cared for at home (Audit Commission 1992).

With the implementation of the community care reforms, nurses now have an additional responsibility in the assessment, and in some cases, the management of greater numbers of needy individuals. Since 1993, local authorities have been responsible for assessing the needs of all people who require social care. These include patients with intractable mental illness discharged into the community, people with learning disabilities previously resident in hospitals, the elderly, the physically disabled and all those in need of residential or nursing home care. Community nurses have an important contribution to make to the care of these patient groups. Depending on local arrangements, they may be required to contribute to health assessment, the arrangement or delivery of care, or the giving of specialist nursing advice (Royal College of Nursing, 1993).

In the context of the expanding role of the community nurse, the need for clinical practice to be underpinned by sound evidence has probably never been more pressing.

The Patient's Charter

The introduction of the internal market in the NHS has brought with it commercially derived language and practices. The very terms 'purchaser' and 'provider' are testimony to this, as is the increasing use of the word 'consumer.' The *Patient's Charter* (Department of Health, 1991b) is an attempt to recognise the rights of service users and illustrates the ideological shift from a passive patient to an active consumer of health care. In addition to identifying what users may expect of the Health Service, the *Patient's Charter* also sets out specific standards of service which will ultimately affect the way community nurses carry out their practice.

Many of the standards of the charter reflect the philosophy which underpins all nursing practice, such as the requirements to respect an individual's privacy, dignity and religious beliefs. Others, like the patient's right to a named nurse responsible for their care, will serve to bring other health professionals into line with how community nurses have always worked.

In contrast to this, the operational standards laid down in the *Patient's Charter*, such as the giving of appointment times and the assurance that all new patients will be seen within a specified time limit, will have an effect on the work of nurses in the community.

These concrete and measurable standards are the ones which will be most binding on community nurses, and which the managers of services will undoubtedly use as an index of the successful deployment of the nursing resource. In these circumstances community nurses will find they are increasingly called upon to account for how they spend their time and to justify the practices and procedures they carry out. The only way they will be able to do this and maintain their own professional standards is by ensuring that wherever possible their practice is founded on sound research based principles.

The Health of the Nation

During the last decade there has been a general realisation that in addition to social and environmental factors and medical interventions, the health of the nation depends just as much on education of the population. The *Health of the Nation* strategy aims to secure improvements in everyone's health by increasing life expectancy and reducing premature death (Department of Health, 1992b). The strategy to minimise the effects of illness or disability, promote healthy lifestyles and improve quality of life will have important consequences for the work of nurses in the community.

Five target areas are identified in the *Health of the Nation*. These target areas include reductions in the incidence of early death from coronary heart disease and stroke, reduced mortality from cancers, accidents, HIV and AIDS and improvement in the quality of life for people with mental illness. As far as community nurses are concerned this implies a substantial increase in their health education activities, in addition to their continuing to care for these patient groups.

With their extensive knowledge of local communities and their accessibility to the general public, community nurses are in a strong position to provide advice and guidance about diet, exercise and healthy living. In addition they can play a pivotal role in prevention of disease and in health screening activities.

In order to justify this expansion of the community nurse's role there is a need to ensure that good practice is underpinned by evidence based guidelines.

Government strategy for nursing, midwifery and health visiting research

The Strategy for Nursing (Department of Health, 1989b) and the Strategy for Nursing Research (Department of Health, 1993) are aiming to ensure that where possible all nursing practice and clinical decisions are research based.

The professional priority is to integrate relevant research into practice at all levels of the Health Service organisation and create a climate in which research is disseminated and utilised by all professional groups. No matter how successful this strategy may be, as far as community nurses are concerned they are the people who will have the ultimate responsibility for applying research to appropriate areas of clinical practice. It is therefore in the best interests of both community nurses and their patients that wherever possible clinical work is founded on solid evidence.

Nursing education initiatives

The Post Registration Education and Practice Project (United Kingdom Central Council for Nursing, Midwifery and Health Visiting, 1991) requires that individual practitioners be accountable for their practices through maintenance of up to date knowl-edge and skills. Personal and professional development is a responsibility of all nurses. Senior community nurses are also going to be taking an increased responsibility for supporting and mentoring their more junior colleagues.

In addition, fundamental changes in basic nurse training realised through the Project 2000 courses (United Kingdom Central Council for Nursing, Midwifery and Health Visiting, 1986), have placed the emphasis squarely on the concept of primary health care and consequently learner nurses are to gain a great deal of their practical clinical experience in community locations.

The advent of Project 2000 implies that community nurses are not only responsible for updating their own practices but also have to find a credible means of transmitting their clinical knowledge to new nurses and ensuring that the clinical practices of the next generation of community nurses are also of the highest standard.

Since the time of the report of the committee on nursing (Department of Health and Social Security 1972) the nursing profession has been striving to develop and consolidate its research base.

Although nursing has been engaged in research activities for over forty years, the relationship between research and practice remains a problem. The dissemination and use of research findings appears to be a difficulty in general nursing (Hockey, 1987) which is compounded in the community. The fact that community nurses are based in clinics, health centres and GP surgeries means they are less likely to have use of resource centres where they can easily access up-to-date clinical information. In addition, much of the work of community nurses is under researched (Luker & Kenrick, 1992). Most clinical studies, particularly those relating to 'technical' practices, have been conducted in the hospital environment and whilst these studies may in principle be relevant to community nursing, in research terms there is nothing to indicate that the findings are transferable. For example, the management of pain in the home presents a very different problem to the community nurse than it does to one working on a hospital ward.

All these changes, together with technological developments in health care, are continually expanding the scope of community nursing practice and increasing the need for community nurses at all levels to have appropriate guidelines to inform all aspects of their clinical work.

ABOUT THIS BOOK

It is against this background that *Clinical Nursing Practice in the Community* has been developed. Although there are many texts which are aimed at community nurses, to date there is no comprehensive reference to clinical procedures which is directed *specifically* at the needs of community nurses and Project 2000 students on community placements.

This book is a direct response to a need for a composite guide to underpin practice. The topics covered in this book have been identified by community nurses themselves, and it has been designed to be useful to both experienced practitioners and new students alike.

Clinical Nursing Practice in the Community is exceptional in that the idea for its compilation emerged from two years of research exploring the mechanisms by which district nurses update their clinical practice (Luker & Kenrick, 1992). The research also identified a need amongst both qualified and student nurses for a handbook of this kind.

The contents have all been described by community nurses as the aspects of their work for which they would most value guidelines for practice. In addition, the format of the text has itself been tested, and found to be the most acceptable and useful way of conveying research information to community nurse practitioners.

Aims of the book

The text aims to provide sound guidance for community nursing practice, with which all community nurses can enhance their clinical skills. Where research evidence exists this is used, but in areas which are under researched the guidance is based on knowledge of cases and professional consensus. The book is not trying be an instruction manual, but rather is gathering together basic information which details the research based principles upon which good practice can be carried out.

Clinical Nursing Practice in the Community is a comprehensive reference work. It acknowledges that individual practitioners will have different levels of expertise and on this basis it is expected that the reader will combine the research based principles outlined with their own experience to adapt to the needs of different clinical situations. The experienced practitioner should also find the text useful as a teaching aid for student nurses.

For the Project 2000 student the text will be a useful practical resource, which together with the support of the professional mentor will supply concrete guidelines upon which good practice can be developed. In addition the references for further reading supplied with each chapter should facilitate the growth of clinical knowledge as the student becomes a more experienced nurse.

Organisation of the text

The contents of this book reflect the changing responsibilities of community nurses. The subjects covered deal with procedures which community nurses identify as being important aspects of their practice, and those which reflect the expansion of the community nurse's role into new areas, in line with policy developments in health care.

The first four chapters of the book deal with areas of clinical care common to everyday practice. These include manual handling of patients, drug administration, nutrition and basic clinical procedures. The next seven chapters then deal with more specific areas of clinical care, where managing the process of care is critical. These include tissue viability and wound care, the management of leg ulcers, the management of pain, promotion of continence, and care of people with hypertension, diabetes and asthma. In the last four chapters long term care is the unifying theme. These chapters include guidance for screening older people, the rehabilitation of patients following stroke, principles of patient education and a chapter on the principles of safe care in the community of the patient with HIV or AIDS.

The chapters are comprehensive in scope and each is intended to stand alone as a reference for its subject matter. The chapter headings describe a broad area of practice and the organisation of the contents arises from the research and reflects the way district nurses conceptualise their clinical work.

The chapters share a similar structure and each consists of background information, guidelines for practice, references for further reading and, where appropriate, practical tools which will be of use to nurses working in the community.

This volume is intended to be useful for all community nurses, and together with the expertise of the reader it is hoped that *Clinical Nursing Practice in the Community* will make an important contribution to the growth of research based practice in the community.

REFERENCES AND FURTHER READING

Audit Commission (1992) *Homeward Bound: A New Course for Community Health* HMSO, London.

Department of Health (1989a) *Working for Patients* HMSO, London

Department of Health (1989b) *A Strategy for Nursing* HMSO, London.

Department of Health (1991a) *Research for Health: a Research and Development Strategy* HMSO, London.

Department of Health (1991b) *The Patients's Charter* HMSO, London.

Department of Health (1992a) *Assessing the Benefits of Health Technologies* HMSO, London.

Department of Health (1992b) *The Health of the Nation* HMSO, London.

Department of Health (1993) *Report of the Taskforce for Research in Nursing, Midwifery and Health Visiting* HMSO, London.

Department of Health and Social Security (1972) *Report of the Committee on Nursing* (the Briggs Report) HMSO, London.

Hockey, L. (1987) Issues in the communication of nursing research *Recent Advances in Nursing: Current Issues* (18) Churchill Livingstone, Edinburgh.

Luker, K.A. & Kenrick, M. (1992) Sources of influence on the clinical decisions of community nurses *Journal of Advanced Nursing* 17, 457–66.

NHS Management Executive (1993) *A Vision for the Future* HMSO, London.

Royal College of Nursing (1993) *Community Care* HMSO/ RCN, London.

United Kingdom Central Council for Nursing, Midwifery and Health Visiting (1986) *Project 2000: a New Preparation for Practice* UKCC, London.

United Kingdom Central Council for Nursing, Midwifery and Health Visiting (1991) *Report of a Proposal for the Future of Community Education and Practice Project* UKCC, London.

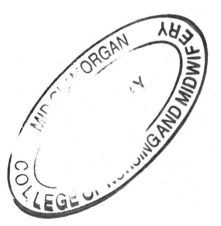

1

Basic Clinical Procedures
Jane Griffiths

1.1 INTRODUCTION

The purpose of this chapter is to provide research based guidance for the commonly performed techniques of eye care, mouth care and venepuncture. The research base for these practices is variable.

Basic procedures for eye care appear to be substantially under–researched; and venepuncture is frequently given no more than passing reference in most nursing and medical textbooks. Mouth care has been researched, but much of the evidence is either contradictory or inconclusive, and the subject does not appear to have made substantial progress since Howarth and Harris published their seminal papers in 1977 and 1980 respectively. Where research evidence is scant, basic principles of anatomy, physiology, pharmacology and bacteriology are used to inform guidance for practice.

1.2 EYE CARE

Despite community nurses' understanding of opthalmics and the relative priority given by them to eye care (Felinski, 1989), there is little empirical data to support the various recommended nursing practices and procedures. Accepted standard principles of eye care are therefore preceded by a detailed look at the anatomy and physiology of the eye, and application of fundamental principles provides a scientific rationale for practice.

Anatomy of the eye

The following description is adapted from Snell (1992).

The Eyeball
The eyeball has three coats which, from the outside in, are the fibrous coat, the vascular pigmented coat and the nervous coat.

Fibrous coat
The fibrous coat is opaque at the back of the eyeball and transparent at the front. The 'posterior' opaque part is the sclera, and the 'anterior' transparent part is the cornea.

The sclera is white and is composed of dense fibrous tissue. The optic nerve leaves it at the lamina cribrosa, which is a weakened area that bulges outwards if there is an increase in intraocular pressure. The sclera is continuous with the cornea, whose principal purpose is the refraction of light. The lens has only a third of the refractive properties of the cornea (Rennie, 1993).

Vascular pigmented coat
The vascular pigmented coat is composed of the choroid, ciliary body and the iris. The ciliary body comprises: the ciliary ring; the ciliary process; and the ciliary muscle. When the ciliary muscle contracts, it pulls the ciliary body forwards, the lens becomes more convex and its refractive power is increased.

The iris is contractile and pigmented with a central aperture, the pupil. It is suspended in aqueous humour and divides the area between the cornea and the lens into the anterior and posterior chambers. It has two types of muscle fibre. Circular muscle constricts the pupil; radial muscle dilates the pupil. The circular muscle is supplied with parasympathetic nerve fibres and the radial muscle by sympathetic nerves.

Nervous coat
The nervous coat is the retina. The optic nerve leaves the retina by the optic disc, also called the 'blind spot' because it has no rod or cone cells.

The eyeball (shown in Fig. 1.1) contains aqueous humour, the vitreous body and the lens.

supports the back of the lens, which is a crystalline, enclosed in a transparent capsule and encircled by the ciliary process. The capsule is constantly under tension as it attempts to change the lens from a disc to a sphere. The circumference of the lens is attached to the ciliary body by a suspensory ligament which keeps the lens flattened to enable focusing on distant objects. To accommodate the eye for close objects the ciliary muscle contracts and the ciliary body is pulled forwards and inwards; the radiating fibres of the ligament are relaxed and the lens becomes more spherical in shape. As a person gets older, the lens

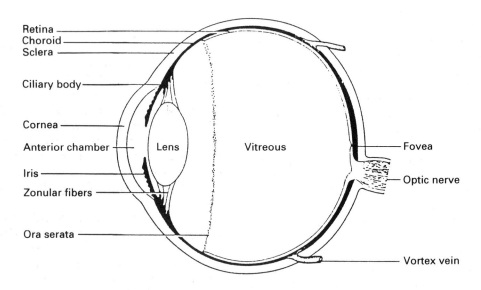

Figure 1.1   The basic structure of the eye. Source: Perry, J.P. and Tullo, A.B. (1993) (eds) *Care of the Ophthalmic Patient*, courtesy of Chapman & Hall Ltd.

Aqueous humour
Aqueous humour is a clear fluid which fills the anterior and posterior chambers. It flows from the posterior chamber to the anterior chamber through the pupil, and is drained away into the canal of Schlemm. Obstruction of the drainage causes glaucoma which leads to degenerative changes and visual impairment. The aqueous humour supports the wall of the eyeball, nourishes the cornea and lens, and removes the products of metabolism.

Vitreous body
The vitreous body is a transparent gel behind the lens. It contributes to the magnifying power of the eye and

becomes denser and less elastic and its ability to accommodate decreases, often necessitating the use of spectacles to focus on close objects.

Eyelids
The eyelids protect the eye from injury and bright light. They are lined with mucous membranes, the conjunctivae. The conjunctivae end where they meet the eyeball at the upper and lower fornices.

Near the medial angle of the eye (nearest to the nose) the eyelashes stop suddenly and there is a small red elevation called the papilla lacrimalis. On this there is a small hole, the punctum lacrimale, through which tears travel down the nose via the canaliculi lacrimales. Tears are produced by the lacrimal gland whose ducts open into the conjunctiva.

Basic physiology of sight

This section relies heavily on the work of Rennie (1993). Light rays are focused onto the retina by the cornea and lens via a process called refraction (bending). In its 'relaxed' elliptical shape, the normal lens will bring distant objects into focus.

To focus on something close, the lens becomes more spherical, increasing the total refractive power of the eye and this is referred to as accommodation. Accommodation is achieved via contraction of the ciliary muscle, which is innervated by parasympathetic nerve fibres. The pupils constrict and the eyes converge on the object. The rays of light once focused on the retina are converted into electrical energy by the photoreceptors, the rods and cones, which connect with other nerve cells in the retina to send the electrical message down the optic nerve. The message travels along nerve pathways to the lateral geniculate body in the brain.

To achieve binocular vision, the nerve fibres from the nasal half of each retina cross over to the other side of the brain at the optic chiasm. Each lateral geniculate body therefore receives nerve fibres from the temporal retina of the corresponding eye and the nasal retina of the opposite eye.

From here the nerve impulse is transmitted to the occipital lobes of the brain where they are formed into an image. The visual cortex, which is within the occipital lobes, is connected to higher centres in the brain, enabling processes such as recognition to occur.

1.3 GUIDANCE FOR PRACTICE – EYE CARE

In the community eye care may be necessary as a pre- or post-operative intervention. It may also be carried out as a treatment for an ophthalmic condition, or to ensure a patient's comfort.

Nurses may have cause to use a variety of topical applications. In addition, they may also be required to demonstrate new techniques to a patient or carer.

Eyedrops

Antibiotics
The epithelium of the cornea is an effective barrier to topical medication, and systemic drugs have considerable difficulty passing from blood to retina or blood to aqueous humour to reach their target. Topical antibiotics such as chloramphenicol are fat soluble, however, and enter the corneal epithelium easily. Chloramphenicol is often prescribed when bacterial infection is suspected (Joyce, 1993) but may have been rendered ineffective by over use (Smith, 1987). Framycetin and neomycin are also in common use.

Anti-inflammatories
Although useful clinically, steroids have side effects. Applied topically or taken systemically, they can lead to glaucoma (Smith, 1987). Intraoccular pressure therefore requires close monitoring in long term use. Topical steroids can also increase susceptibility to bacterial, viral and fungal infection (Joyce, 1993).

Prednisolone, betamethosone and dexamethasone are in common use. Prednisolone may be combined with an antibiotic such as neomycin as in Predsol N. Like systemic steroids, topical steroids should not be stopped suddenly.

As an alternative to steroids, topical indomethacin is increasingly prescribed to prevent inflammation following cataract surgery (Joyce, 1993).

Antihistamines are primarily for the treatment of conjunctivits caused by allergens. Sodium cromglycate, a mast cell stabilizer, is one example.

Drugs acting on the sympathetic and parasympathetic nervous system
Mydriatic eyedrops achieve pupil dilation or mydriasis by either stimulating the sympathetic receptors in the iris or blocking the parasympathetic (cholinergic) receptors. This is useful for examination of the eye.

Miotic eyedrops achieve pupil constriction or miosis by blocking the sympathetic receptors or stimulating the parasympathetic receptors. This can be useful in the treatment of glaucoma, with the narrowed pupil assisting aqueous drainage.

The beta-blocking eyedrop timolol is useful in glaucoma because it reduces aqueous secretion, but over liberal dosage may lead to bradycardia, heart failure or asthma in the susceptible, as it enters the blood stream via puncta lacrimale and canaliculi lacrimales. It is therefore contraindicated where these conditions co-exist (Smith, 1987).

Lubricants

Where dry eye is present due to disease, radiotherapy or reduced blink reflex, artificial tears such as hypromellose or methylcellulose can be helpful (Pritchard & Mallett, 1993).

Instilling eyedrops

The following strictly aseptic procedure is recommended for the instillation of eyedrops (Corrin, 1993):

- Check the bottles and dosages, and for which eye the drop is prescribed. A patient may need a miotic in one eye in preparation for extraction of cataract, and a mydriatic in the other for the treatment of glaucoma.
- Ask the patient to lie or sit down with head well supported and in good light.
- If the eye is discharging and swabbing is required, sterile swabs soaked in saline should be used. The motion is from the inner to the outer aspect of the eye. Cleaning the lower lid is performed with the patient looking up; the upper lid is cleaned with the eyes closed. Each swab should be used once only.
- Hold a dry sterile swab below the lower lid, slightly everting it.
- Ask the patient to look up so that the eyedrop can be instilled into the lower fornix of the conjunctiva and not onto the highly sensitive cornea.
- Hold the bottle sufficiently close to the eye to ensure accuracy and comfort, but sufficiently far way to avoid contamination of the dropper: about 1 cm or 0.5 inch. The drop should not be dropped from a great height onto the sensitive cornea.
- Instil one drop into the lower fornix between the middle and outer third of the eye.
- Ask the patient to close the eyes. Wipe the area gently to absorb any excess solution which might irritate the skin.

If ointment is prescribed, the eyes should be closed and the ointment applied in a stream along the lid margins. It should then be spread gently and evenly with a sterile swab. Alternatively it may be inserted into the lower fornix in a stream from the inner to the outer aspect (Corrin, 1993).

Problems specific to community nursing

Although the instillation of eyedrops, particularly post operatively, can form a substantial proportion of community nursing work (Williams & Winfield 1990), its importance may be undervalued by some community nurses (Felinski, 1989). This is perhaps because for several weeks following surgery for cataract extraction, for example, insertion of eyedrops may be required up to four times a day. This places tremendous pressure on an already overstretched community nursing service, and keeping to any regular time for the visits can be almost impossible (Felinski, 1989).

The answer lies in teaching either the patients themselves or carers to carry out the procedure. But research has shown that self care in eye medication remains for many an elusive ideal, with problems ranging from touching the eye with the dropper to difficulties in aiming the drop in the correct place (Burns & Mulley, 1992).

In many cases it will be possible to teach someone else to instill the eye drops safely. According to one survey, this still leaves about a third of patients for whom it may not be practicable to enlist the help of a relative, friend or neighbour (Felinski, 1989). Yet too few patients appear to be offered devices to assist in the instillation of eyedrops (Burns & Mulley, 1992), a measure which demonstrably improves the accuracy of eyedrop administration (Williams & Winfield, 1990).

Where a preparation is available as an ointment this may be preferred to a drop if the drug needs to stay in contact with the eye for a longer period. However, the temporary clouding of vision caused by ointments may be a hazard for a patient living alone.

Aids to self care

Williams and Winfield (1990) found that one of the more commonly used compliance aids, the cut away eyebath, was unmanageable for some patients. Squeezing the bottle was a problem, as was taking the cap off without contaminating the dropper. They therefore designed the Opticare, which in trials with persons aged 60 and over successfully delivered the drop in the correct place for 49% at the first attempt and 63% at the second attempt. Trials in the community were equally successful even in arthritic patients. All 14 patients surveyed had experienced difficulty in administering drops. Only one could not manage the device, and three required extra time for teaching to avoid over application.

Post operative complications

The majority of eye patients seen by the community nurse are likely to have had cataract extraction (Perry, 1993). With shorter hospital stays and a lot more day case surgery (Bloomfield, 1990; Traynar, 1990; Morris, 1993), it is vital that the community nurse recognises basic post operative complications so that the patient can be referred back to the hospital without delay (Perry, 1993). Both eyes should be examined for the purpose of comparison. In good light using a pen torch look for the following possible complications:

- Hyphaemea: blood in the anterior chamber, which presents as a dark area at the bottom of the iris.
- Hypopyon: white blood cells in the anterior chamber, which presents as a white area at the bottom of the iris.
- Leaking wound.
- Prolapsed iris.
- Corneal oedema.

Any of these can occur if the eye is rubbed or knocked. An eye shield is therefore recommended at night.

Poor vision is not a complication of eye surgery: return to good vision should not be expected for several weeks. Deterioration of vision or an increase in pain are complications, however, and the patient should be referred back to the hospital.

Self care
Although the patient should have received individualised care instructions prior to discharge from hospital, the following general advice should be followed (Bloomfield, 1990):

- Avoid heavy lifting, including shopping.
- Avoid straining as a result of constipation: a mild laxative may be prescribed.
- Rest – do not resume heavy physical work until advised by the hospital and avoid excessive coughing.

Home environment
Patients who are visually impaired for reasons other than the immediate after effect of cataract extraction can benefit from the following changes to the home environment:

- Windows should be clean and net curtains removed to allow maximum natural light into the room. Curtains that tie back or blinds that can be pulled down are useful to reduce the intermittent glare of sunlight.
- Fluorescent lighting or reading lamps are useful because they do not create shadows. Light switches should be sited so that they can be switched on before the person enters the room. Exterior lights are helpful as are security lights.
- Room lights can be placed strategically in areas where specific tasks are carried out. Light bulbs should be of the maximum safe wattage.
- Lampshades should be positioned to direct the light into the right place.
- Colour contrasts are helpful: door frames painted to stand out from a pale wall; pale unpatterned carpets; steps with white edges. In any area of the house, it is useful to have contrasting colours: toilet rolls, pans, cutlery, razors that stand out against their background (Perry, 1993).

1.4 EYE CARE SUMMARY

Despite the important part vision plays in everyday life, interestingly there has been very little nursing research into aspects of eye care. Community nurses are regularly involved in eye care procedures, most commonly as a pre-operative or post-operative intervention.

The installation of eye drops or other topical applications is a regular feature of community nursing work. When possible the community nurse teaches the patient or carer to undertake the intervention; however, it has to be recognised that this is not always possible, especially with elderly people.

The mechanics of eye care in the community can prove difficult. The frequency of the application of the medication may mean that the nurse has to visit up to three times a day and this is difficult to fit into a busy schedule. Finally, many more patients could be taught to meet their own eye care requirements if the procedure was not so reliant on good manual dexterity. More effort needs to be directed towards the production of user friendly devices. This might be possible if nurses and manufacturers were prepared to work together.

1.5 MOUTH CARE

Mouth care is arguably one of the most basic and important yet undervalued and overlooked of all nursing procedures (Shepherd *et al.*, 1987; Crosby, 1989; Boyle, 1992). In a much publicised study, Howarth (1977) wrote that mouth care practice has 'remained virtually unchanged over many years', an observation which has been echoed repeatedly over subsequent decades (Harris, 1980; MacMillan, 1981; Gibbons, 1983; Shepherd *et al.*, 1987; Crosby, 1989; Barnett, 1991; Holmes & Mountain, 1993).

Mouth care procedures in the community are no different from those practised anywhere else. Particularly with the emphasis on individualised assessment, the standard mouth care pack is almost obsolete (Jenkins, 1989). The main issues for community nursing would appear to be patient education and education of the carers who carry out mouth care. Except perhaps in terminal care, mouth care is increasingly unlikely to be carried out by a trained nurse (Boyle, 1992). Although there are caveats in the literature on mouth care (Trenter-Roth & Creason, 1986; Boyle, 1992), there is now an adequate if not exhaustive body of research on which to build safe and effective guidance for practice.

Indications

Mouth care is important for all patients. Poor oral health and the need for increased attention to mouth care is likely to be indicated where:

- a patient is taking little in the way of food and fluids (Howarth, 1977).
- there is xerostoma (dry mouth) due to an underlying pathology which decreases salivary production, e.g. Sjogren's syndrome, which is common in older women (MacDonald & Marino, 1992).
- there is drug induced decrease in saliva production, e.g. by morphine (White *et al.*, 1989), or anticholinergics, anti-depressants, anti-histamines, anti-Parkinsons agents, anti-hypertensives, beta-blockers (McDonald & Marino, 1992).
- the patient has undergone chemotherapy or radiotherapy resulting in both dry mouth and stomatitis (Daeffler 1980a).
- there has been a decrease in manual dexterity due to arthritis or a decrease in motivation for self care due, for example, to depression, confusion or dementia (Redfern, 1991).
- There is gingivitis caused by the build up of plaque (Pope *et al.*, 1975).

There are also psychosocial implications of poor oral health (Trenter-Roth & Creason, 1986). The mouth plays an important role in both verbal and non–verbal communication: a dry mouth may cause problems with speech, and dry lips will crack with facial expression. Halitosis can be socially isolating.

Anatomy and physiology

This section draws upon the work of Snell (1992), Ganong (1989) and Vander *et al.*, (1979).

The mouth is subdivided into the vestibule which lies between the lips and cheeks externally and the gums and teeth internally; and the mouth cavity proper which lies within the alveolar arches, gums and teeth. The adult mouth has 32 permanent teeth.

The cheek forms the lateral wall of the vestibule. It is composed of the buccinator muscle and is lined with mucous membrane. Opposite the second molar tooth is an opening in the mucous membrane of the duct of one of three salivary glands, the parotid.

The mouth proper has a roof which is divided into the hard palate in front and the soft palate behind. The soft palate is continuous with the lateral wall of the pharynx, which is the entrance to the oesophagus. The wall of the pharynx has three layers: mucous, fibrous and muscular. In front of the pharynx is the larynx (voice box) which is the entrance to the trachea. It has a glottis which is the opening between the vocal chords. The epiglottis is a flap of elastic cartilage and mucous membrane, which covers the closed glottis during swallowing.

The floor of the mouth is formed by the tongue and

the membrane attaching the tongue to the mandible. The tongue is muscular, well innervated and covered with mucous membrane. The midline of the membrane is the frenulum which connects the underside of the tongue to the floor of the mouth. The duct of the submandibular salivary gland opens from a papilla at the side of the frenulum. From the papilla, a ridge of mucous membrane formed by the sublingual salivary gland extends backwards. The ridge is called the sublingual fold. The ducts of the sublingual salivary gland open onto the sublingual fold.

Saliva

Saliva is 99% water. The rest is composed mainly of proteins called mucins which when chemically bonded to water produce highly viscous mucous. The presence of food or something acidic in the mouth increases the rate of salivary production. Each day one to two litres of saliva are secreted, which highlights the need for adequate fluid intake. The functions of saliva are to:

- facilitate swallowing;
- keep the mouth moist;
- act as a solvent for molecules that stimulate the taste buds;
- aid speech by facilitating the movement of the lips and tongue;
- keep the mouth and teeth clean.

Saliva may also have some bactericidal activity. If saliva production is reduced for any reason, all of these functions will be affected.

Swallowing

Once food has been masticated by the teeth and lubricated by saliva, the resulting bolus is forced to the back of the mouth by the tongue. It moves into the pharynx and the soft palate rises to seal off the nasal cavity. The larynx rises and closes the glottis to prevent food from entering the trachea. The bolus tilts the epiglottis backwards to cover the closed glottis. Breathing stops momentarily while the skeletal muscle of the upper part of the oesophagus contracts, and the hypopharyngeal sphincter opens to allow the bolus to pass. Once the bolus has passed, the muscles relax, the sphincter closes, the glottis opens and breathing recommences. Peristalsis, rather than gravity, forces the bolus towards the stomach.

1.6 GUIDANCE FOR PRACTICE – MOUTH CARE

According to Pope *et al.* (1975), Allbright (1984) and Pritchard & Mallett (1993) the interrelated aims of mouth care are as follows:

- patient comfort and reduction in pain;
- oral hygiene;
- to keep oral mucosa moist;
- to prevent plaque build up, dental decay and infections;
- to increase the appetite.

Assessment

The following areas should be assessed in all patients:

- Ability to carry out mouth care (physically/level of understanding)
- Motivation
- Nutritional status
- Fluid intake
- Medication (including chemotherapy).

Where a patient is assessed to be at risk of poor oral health observation of the mouth should be carried out in good light using a pen torch. The following areas should be assessed:

- Health of gums
- Condition of teeth
- Condition and fit of dentures
- Colour and texture of tongue
- Condition of mucous membranes
- Condition of lips
- Oral pain
- Swallowing reflex
- Voice/speech
- Consistency and quantity of saliva.

Procedures for mouth care are shown in Table 1.1.

Oral assessment guides

Several oral assessment guides (OAGs) have been developed, are gaining in popularity and are frequently recommended in the literature. The importance of OAGs from a research point of view is that

Table 1.1 Summary of mouth care procedure.

- The nurse should wear gloves to minimise the risk of cross infection, including the risk of coming into contact with blood.
- Fluoride toothpaste and a soft paediatric sized toothbrush or electric toothbrush should be used.
- Brushing should include the teeth, tongue, gums and oral tissues.
- Unless there is stomatitis, interdental cleaning can be carried out using waxed floss.
- Teeth should be brushed in individual strokes away from the gums.
- To remove plaque and debris from the gingival margin the toothbrush should be placed at an angle of 45° and agitated with a small vibratory movement.
- The mouth should then be rinsed with water, or a chlorhexidine mouthwash if infection is present.

they can produce baseline data from which the various techniques for mouth care can be assessed.

Holmes and Mountain (1993) evaluated three OAGs for reliability, validity and clinical usefulness: those of Passos and Brand (1966), Beck (1979) and Eilers *et al.* (1988). Each guide assessed the lips, tongue, mucous membranes, gingiva (gums) and swallowing reflex. In addition, the Passos and Brand (1966) OAG assessed the palate, and the other two the teeth and voice.

Although Holmes and Mountain (1993) found one of the OAGs (Eilers et al., 1988) comprehensive and easy to use, they found that all three guides were of questionable reliability and validity. The guides were useful for the detection of gross abnormalities, but there were several important omissions from each, particularly in relation to pain, food consumption and changes in taste sensation.

Another OAG is the risk assessment guide of Jenkins (1989) which, although it was developed for use in ITU, Redfern (1991) recommends for oral assessment of the elderly. The problem with this guide for use in the community is that the maximum recommended time interval between episodes of mouth care is two hours. This is impractical without the willing assistance of trained carers, but does highlight the fact that mouth care in the critically ill should be performed frequently.

Mouth care preparations

Mouth care preparations are many and varied, but few are now recognised to have any therapeutic value (Trenter-Roth & Creason, 1986). One of the problems with assessing products is that without a standardised oral assessment guide, there are no baseline data from which to compare one product

with another. Evidence to support or refute the efficacy of some of the more commonly used preparations is presented below:

Lemon and glycerine
Lemon and glycerine is used increasingly less these days because it has no established therapeutic value, and the acidity of the lemon may be destructive to the tooth enamel of dentate patients (Trenter-Roth & Creason, 1986; Crosby, 1989). In theory, the natural acidity of the lemon stimulates salivation, but this effect is sometimes short lasting (Howarth, 1977). Evidence for the hydrating effects of glycerine is contradictory: whether it attracts water to or repels water from the oral mucosa remains unclear.

Hydrogen peroxide
Although in theory freshly prepared hydrogen peroxide solution debrides the mouth mechanically (Shepherd *et al.*, 1987) there is no conclusive research evidence to support its continued use (Trenter-Roth & Creason, 1986). Although it may have some bactericidal effect (Passos & Brand, 1966), claims that the liberation of oxygen can inhibit the growth of anaerobic bacteria may be unfounded if, as is recommended, the solution is rinsed away with warm water or saline to minimise the risk of irritation (Pritchard & Mallett, 1993).

Sodium bicarbonate
Sodium bicarbonate has a similar effervescent action to hydrogen peroxide, although it has an unpleasant taste which precludes its use in some patients. In too strong a solution, the alkalinity which might otherwise exert a mild bactericidal effect, can damage the oral mucosa (Passos & Brand, 1966). It may, however, be useful in stomatitis associated with cancer chemotherapy in a solution of one 5 ml teaspoon to

500 ml of water (Daeffler, 1980a; Allbright, 1984; Crosby, 1989).

Chlorhexidine
Of all the bactericides available in proprietary mouthwashes, chlorhexidine appears to have the greatest therapeutic value in reducing bacteria and the formation of plaque (Crosby, 1989). It is recommended as a useful adjunct to brushing and flossing in the infected mouth, but also prophylactically in the mouth care of patients undergoing chemotherapy (Crosby, 1989). It is also available as a gel. Chlorhexidine may, however, stain the teeth of dentate patients in long term use (Trenter-Roth & Creason, 1986).

Analgesic preparations
In mild stomatitis, and if the initial stinging sensation is tolerated, an analgesic mouthwash or gel is recommended. When pain is severe, systemic analgesia is the preferred treatment (Allbright, 1984). Topical or systemic analgesics will, however, reduce sensitivity to potentially hazardous hot food and drink (Daeffler, 1980a).

Salivary substitutes
Salivary substitutes may be useful in xerostoma. They usually contain carboxymethylcellulose and are recommended for use before retiring at night (Daeffler, 1980b; MacDonald & Marino, 1992).

Saline/tap water
Unless it is sterile, the advantage of normal saline over tap water has yet to be established. In the absence of research evidence to support the use of more expensive products, plain water is recommended for rinsing the uninfected mouth (Gooch, 1985). It is non-irritant and rehydrating and may be the most important constituent of commercial mouthwashes, bearing in mind that saliva is 99% water (Trenter-Roth & Creason, 1986).

Toothpaste
There is now substantial evidence from dental research of the efficacy of brushing the teeth with fluoride toothpastes. It is the treatment of choice in the mouth care of the dentate patient who has no evidence of stomatitis (Trenter-Roth & Creason, 1986; O'Hare, 1991; Richardson, 1987). Toothpaste should be rinsed out because some of the ingredients might dry the oral mucosa.

Yellow soft paraffin
Vaseline or yellow soft paraffin is popular, effective and non-irritant. It is recommended for use on dry and cracked lips (Daeffler, 1980a; Shepherd et al., 1987).

Tools for mouth care
A soft paediatric sized toothbrush is the preferred tool for mouth care because it is familiar, effective in the removal of debris and plaque, liked by patients and easily available (Howarth, 1977; Harris, 1980; Trenter-Roth & Creason, 1986; Crosby, 1989). An equally suitable choice is the electric toothbrush (Harris, 1980). Toothbrushes should be used for brushing the tongue, oral mucosa and gums as well as the teeth (Ettinger & Manderson, 1975).

A swabbed finger is another popular alternative (Harris, 1980) which may be preferred in the endentelous patient or where there is stomatitis and brushing cannot be tolerated.

The foam stick has been found to be an acceptable and comfortable tool for mouth care, although its effectiveness in removing plaque is questionable (Howarth, 1977; Harris, 1980).

Forceps are expensive and unwieldy and their continued use cannot be justified (Howarth, 1977; Harris, 1980).

Specific problems

Dentures
Dentures should be checked for general condition and fit. They should be washed in warm water and a non-abrasive product such as soap, detergent or one of the proprietary cleaners. They should be soaked overnight in water or a proprietary soaking solution to prevent them from drying out and warping (Clarke, 1993). Where a patient has infected stomatitis, dentures should be removed for periods during the day, as well as at night, and soaked in chlorhexidine.

Gingivitis (inflammation of the gums)
Healthy gums are pink. One of the major causes of gingivitis is the build up of plaque at the gingival margin. The gums will be deep red/bluish, inflamed, will bleed easily and often recede. The teeth are sometimes loose. A dental referral for removal of calculus is required followed by correct brushing to remove plaque (Pope et al., 1975).

Stomatitis

Stomatitis is an unavoidable complication of the non-discriminatory cytotoxicity of chemotherapy. A toothbrush is unlikely to be tolerated (Daeffler, 1980b), so a swabbed finger can be used. Sodium bicarbonate is also recommended (Daeffler, 1980a; Richardson, 1987). Analgesic/anaesthetic mouthwashes can be helpful in mild stomatitis but systemic analgesia will be required if the pain is severe.

Specific infections

Where there is persistent infection of the mouth, the organism responsible should be identified by sending a swab to the pathology laboratory for culture and sensitivity. Specific antimicrobial medication should be commenced as soon as possible.

Problems specific to the community

Although patients should be encouraged to carry out mouth care for themselves, there will be circumstances when this is not possible. When carers are attending to patients' general hygiene needs, it is important that they are taught the principles of mouth care.

A recent study found that elderly persons in the community may find it difficult to get to a dentist (Fox, 1992). For these patients, it is worth finding out which local dentists will visit the home. The endentelous patient should still visit the dentist to have prostheses checked for cracks and fit.

1.7 MOUTH CARE SUMMARY

Mouth care is important for all people. Poor oral health is most likely when a patient is taking little in the way of food and fluids or where there is a dry mouth due to underlying pathology or drugs.

Several oral assessment guides (Holmes & Mountain, 1993) have been developed. These have been found to be useful for the detection of gross abnormalities, but there are a number of omissions from each particularly in relation to pain, food consumption and changes in taste sensation.

Mouth care preparations are many and varied and few have been shown to have any real therapeutic value. The treatment of choice in the care of dentate patients is brushing the teeth and gums with fluoride toothpaste. In edentulous patients it is also possible to brush the gums, oral mucosa and tongue; a soft paediatric toothbrush is best for this purpose.

Mouth care is a simple procedure. It is important because if well done it can contribute greatly to patient comfort.

1.8 VENEPUNCTURE

Community nurses are increasingly required to carry out venepuncture, a routine clinical procedure for obtaining specimens of blood for haematological, bacteriological or biochemical analysis. Where research into venepuncture exists, it has tended to focus on setting up and monitoring intravenous infusions (Hecker 1988). There is little research on the technique of venepuncture *per se*, although data are available on the way in which techniques affect test results (Leppanen, 1988; Greenland et al., 1990; McMullan *et al.*, 1990). This, plus anatomy, physiology and bacteriology is used to inform safe practice.

Selection of site

Although very occasionally the veins of the lower limb are used for venepuncture this is unlikely to be safe practice in the community where a high percentage of patients are elderly and housebound. Trauma to the veins of the leg could result in ulceration or phlebitis if any underlying pathology is present.

It is recommended that the veins of the upper limb (Fig. 1.2) are used, namely branches of the basilic vein, cephalic vein and median cubital vein in the antecubital fossa. Pollard (1990) recommends that if venepuncture is carried out in the antecubital fossa, there is least risk of damaging corresponding nerves and arteries accidentally, because they are protected in this region by the bicipital aponeurosis. For ease of specimen collection, when selecting veins outside the antecubital fossa, junctions in the venous network should be avoided and if possible, the needle should be inserted above the valve.

(a)

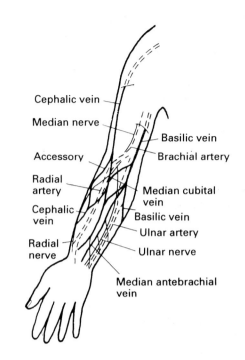

(b)

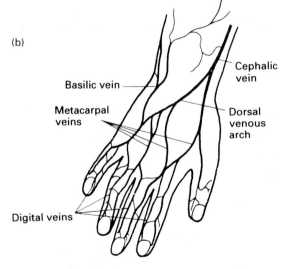

Figure 1.2 Veins of the hand and forearm: (a) superficial veins of the forearm; (b) superficial veins of the dorsal aspect of the hand. Source: *The Royal Marsden Hospital Manual of Clinical Nursing Procedures* (3rd edn), Pritchard & Mallett, Blackwell Science Ltd.

The middle layer of the vein wall is the tunica media. It is muscular and innervated with sympathetic nerve fibres. Ideally the vein will be dilated and either visible or palpable prior to venepuncture. When a patient is anxious, cold or dehydrated, the veins are likely to be more difficult to locate. The physical trauma of inserting a needle into the vein can cause it to collapse or go into a spasm. Factors which will cause vasodilation are warmth, mechanical stimulation (gently tapping or stroking the vein) and local application of the vasodilator glyceryl trinitrate, if medically prescribed for this purpose.

Sites to avoid

If a vein is sclerosed, fibrosed, thrombosed or tortuous, it should be avoided for venepuncture. Likewise veins that are fine and fragile or obviously inflamed. A healthy vein feels soft and springy and will empty and refill again on palpation.

Where there is underlying pathology or injury, the veins may not be suitable for venepuncture. An arm that has been affected by a cerebrovascular accident should be avoided, or if there has been a partial amputation. Fractured limbs, lymphodaematous or oedematous limbs should be avoided.

1.9 GUIDANCE FOR PRACTICE – VENEPUNCTURE

Although blood cultures themselves are unlikely to become contaminated during venepuncture (Shahar *et al.*, 1990), the procedure should be conducted with strict asepsis because both the skin and the circulatory system are breached by the needle, allowing potential pathogens to enter. Handwashing and the use of strong latex gloves protects the nurse from contamination from blood products, and the patient from bacterial contamination from the nurse's hands. Skin flora can still be introduced, however, if the patient's skin is not properly cleaned. The basic procedure for venepuncture is as follows.

Equipment

Where possible, in order to minimise the risk of contact with blood products and needle stick injury, the Vacutainer system for specimen collection is recommended. Equipment required for venepuncture is:

- tourniquet or sphygmomanometer and cuff;
- sterile alcohol prepared cleansing swab;
- vacuum specimen tube holder if using the Vacutainer system;
- a needle designed for the Vacutainer system (19 or 21 gauge);
- small sterile gauze pads or cotton wool balls;
- small plaster or surgical tape;
- protective surgical gloves;
- colour coded bottles;
- specimen requisition form;
- sharps disposal bin.

If not using the Vacutainer system a syringe large enough to accommodate the volume of blood and a 21 gauge needle are required. The risk with using finer needles is that there is increased likelihood either of the blood clotting before it is transferred to the bottles, or of haemolysis (damage to red blood cells).

A winged infusion device (butterfly with adapter) is recommended if a large sample of blood is required from any site other than the antecubital fossa, or if blood is to be taken from an awkward site such as a small vein in the wrist (Millam, 1985).

Procedure for taking blood

- Seat the patient comfortably in adequate light with arm supported to allow maximum extension of the elbow.
- Place a tourniquet above the elbow and antecubital fossa and inspect for a suitable vein either visually or by palpation. If no vein is obvious, try any of the following:
  - instead of a tourniquet inflate a sphygmomanometer cuff to a pressure between systolic and diastolic;
  - gently tap or rub the arm;
  - instruct patient to squeeze the hand open and closed;
  - apply a hot compress or soak the arm in hot water.
- When a suitable vein has been chosen clean the skin with the alcohol swab for at least 30 seconds and allow it to dry (to minimise stinging).
- With one hand gently stretch the skin over the

vein about 2 cm below the proposed insertion site.
- With the other hand insert the needle with bevel uppermost into the vein at an angle of 45° with the arm. Once flashback of blood has occurred the needle can be levelled off slightly.
- If using the Vacutainer system, the bottle will automatically fill. Depending on which tests are required, detach the bottle and attach appropriate bottles until filled.
- If using a needle and syringe steady the syringe with one hand and pull back the plunger with the other until the required amount of blood is collected.
- Release the tourniquet, place cotton wool over site of entry and withdraw the needle.
- When the needle is withdrawn, apply pressure to the point of entry for two to three minutes with the arm held straight (Dyson & Bogod, 1987). If a syringe is used, ask the patient to apply pressure while blood is transferred to the bottles. Do not release pressure until haemostasis has occurred (Godwin et al., 1992). A straight arm and pressure sustained until haemostasis reduces the risk of bruising.
- Apply a plaster to the arm or tape on a cotton wool ball.
- Dispose of the syringe and needle in the sharps container without recapping (Reed, 1987).

If during a difficult venepuncture the vein balloons under the skin, do not persevere. The needle should be removed and pressure applied to the site, followed by a sterile dressing.

Elderly patients
In the older person, superficial veins on the arm are often threadlike and fragile. It is worth palpating for deeper veins. If a fragile vein must be used, a smaller gauged needle is less likely to collapse the vein, although the risk of haemolysis is increased.

Transporting blood
When transporting clotted samples, care should be taken not to lie the bottle on its side or the blood will clot along the sides of the bottle and not in a uniform plug at the bottom.

1.10 VENEPUNCTURE SUMMARY

It is becoming commonplace for community nurses to carry out venepuncture. There is very little research concerning the technique itself, however the way the venepuncture is carried out may ultimately influence the test results. Although blood cultures are unlikely to become contaminated during venepuncture, the procedure should be conducted with strict asepsis.

1.11 REFERENCES AND FURTHER READING

Eye care

Bloomfield, L. (1990) Day case cataracts, *Journal of District Nursing*, February, 5–6.

Burns, E., Mulley, G.P. (1991) Practical problems with eyedrops among elderly ophthalmology eye patients, *Age and Aging*, 21, 168–70.

Corrin, L. (1993) Principles of inpatient care. In *Care of the Ophthalmic Patient* (Ed. by J.P. Perry & A.B. Tullo) Chapman and Hall, London.

Donnelly, D. (1987) Instilling eyedrops: difficulties experienced by patients following cataract surgery, *Journal of Advanced Nursing*, 12, 235–43.

Felinski, S. (1989) Not seeing eye to eye, *Nursing Times*, May 17, **85**, 20, 57–9.

Joyce, P.W. (1993) Pharmacology. In *Care of the Ophthalmic Patient* (Ed. by J.P. Perry & A.B. Tullo) Chapman and Hall, London.

Morris, R. (1993) Advances in cataract surgery, *The Practitioner*, June, 237, 502–6.

Perry, J.P. (1993) Aspects of community care. In *Care of the Ophthalmic Patient* (Ed. by J.P. Perry & A.B. Tullo) Chapman and Hall, London.

Pritchard, A.P. and Mallett, J. (1993) *The Royal Marsden Manual of Clinical Nursing Procedures*, 3rd Edition, Blackwell Science Ltd, Oxford.

Rennie, I. (1993) Examination of the eye. In *Care of the Ophthalmic Patient* (Ed. by J.P. Perry & A.B. Tullo) Chapman and Hall, London.

Smith, S. (1987) Drugs and the eye, *Nursing Times*, June 24, **83**, 25, 48–50.

Snell, R.S. (1992) *Clinical Anatomy for Medical Students* 4th edition, Little, Brown and Company, Boston, USA.

Traynar, M. (1990) Day case eye surgery, *Nursing Times*, September 26, **86**, 39, 54–6.

Williams, A. & Winfield, A. (1990) Topical medication for eye patients, *Nursing Times*, July 4, **86**, 27, 42–3.

Mouth care

Allbright, A. (1984) Oral care for the cancer chemotherapy patient, *Nursing Times*, May 23, 40–42.

Barnett, J. (1991) A reassessment of oral health care, *Professional Nurse*, September, 703–8.

Beck, S. (1979) Impact of a systemic oral care protocol on stomatitis after chemotherapy, *Cancer Nursing*, **2**, 3, 185–9.

Boyle, S. (1992) Assessing mouth care, *Nursing Times*, April 8, **88**, 15, 44–6.

Clarke, G. (1993) Mouth care and the hospitalised patient, *British Journal of Nursing*, **2**, 4, 225–7.

Crosby, C. (1989) Method in mouth care, *Nursing Times*, August 30, **85**, 35, 38–41.

Daeffler, R. (1980a) Oral hygiene measures for patients with cancer 1, *Cancer Nursing*, October, 345–56.

Daeffler, R. (1980b) Oral hygiene measures for patients with cancer 2, *Cancer Nursing*, December, 427–32.

Eilers, J., Berger, A.M. & Petersen, M.C. (1988) Development testing and application of the oral assessment guide, *Oncology Nursing Forum*, **15**, 3, 325–30.

Ettinger, R.L., Manderson, R.D. (1975) Dental care of the elderly, *Nursing Times*, June 26, 1003–1006.

Fox, L. (1992) The tooth of the matter, *Journal of Community Nursing*, June, 16–17.

Ganong, W.F. (1989) *Review of Medical Physiology*. Lang Medical Publications, Los Altos, California.

Gibbons, D.E. (1983) Mouth care procedures, *Nursing Times*, February 16, 30.

Gooch, J. (1985) Mouthcare, *Professional Nurse*. December, 77–8.

Harris, M.D. (1980) Tools for mouth care, *Nursing Times*, February 21, 340–42.

Holmes, S. & Mountain, E. (1993) Assessment of oral health status: evaluation of three oral assessment guides, *Journal of Clinical Nursing*, **2**, 35–40.

Howarth, H. (1977) Mouth care procedures for the very ill, *Nursing Times*, March 10, 354–5.

Jenkins, D. (1989) Oral care in ICU: an important nursing role, *Nursing Standard*, **4**, 7, 24–8.

MacDonald, E. & Marino, C. (1992) Dry mouth: common but treatable, *Geriatric Medicine*, June, 43–9.

MacMillan, K. (1981) New goals for oral hygiene, *The Canadian Nurse*, March 40–3.

O'Hare, A. (1991) Dental Health, *Journal of District Nursing*, April, 4–6.

Passos, J.Y. & Brand, I.M. (1966) Effects of agents used for oral hygiene, *Nursing Research*, 15, 196–202.

Pope, W., Reitz, M., Patrick, M. (1975) A study of oral hygiene in the geriatric patient, *International Journal of Nursing Studies*, 12, 65–92.

Pritchard, A.P. & Mallett, M. (1993) *Royal Marsden Manual of Clinical Nursing Procedures* 3rd Edition, Blackwell Scientific, Oxford.

Redfern, S. (1991) *Nursing Elderly People*, Churchill Livingstone, Edinburgh.

Richardson, A. (1987) A process standard for oral care, *Nursing Times*, **83**, 32, 38–40.

Shepherd, G., Page, C. & Sammon, P. (1987) The mouth trap, *Nursing Times*, May 13, **83**, 19, 24–7.

Snell, R.S. (1992) *Clinical Anatomy for Medical Students*, 4th Edition, Little, Brown and Company, Boston, USA.

Trenter-Roth, P. & Creason, N.S. (1986) Nurse administered oral hygiene: is there a scientific basis, *Journal of Advanced Nursing*, 11, 3, 323–31.

Vander, A.J., Sherman, J.H. & Luciano, D.S. (1979) *The Mechanism of Body Function*. Tata MacGraw Hill Publishing Company Ltd, New Dehli.

White, I.D., Hoskin, P.J., Hanks, G.W. & Bliss, J.M. (1989) *British Medical Journal*, May 6, **298**, 1222–3.

Venepuncture

Dyson, A., Bogod, D. (1987) Minimizing bruising in the antecubital fossa after venepuncture, *British Medical Journal*, June 27, **294**, 1659.

Godwin, P.G.R., Cuthbert, A.C. & Choyce, A. (1992) Reducing bruising after venepuncture, *Quality in Health Care*, **1**, 245–6.

Greenland, P., Bowley, N.L., Meiklejohn, B., Doane, K.L. & Sparks C.E. (1990) Blood cholesterol concentration: fingerstick plasma versus venous serum sampling, *Clinical Chemistry*, **4**, 36, 628–30.

Hecker, J. (1988) Improved technique in intravenous therapy, *Nursing Times*, August 24, **84**, 34, 28–33.

Leppanen, E.A. (1988) Experimental basis of standardised specimen collection: the effect of the site of venepuncture on the blood picture, the white blood cell differential count and the serum albumin concentration, *European Journal of Haematology*, **41**, 445–8.

McMullan, A.D., Burns, J. & Paterson, C.R. (1990) Venepuncture for calcium assays: should we still avoid the tourniquet? *Postgraduate Medical Journal*, **66**, 547–8.

Millam, D.A. (1985) How to get into hard to stick veins, *Registered Nurse*, April, 34–5.

Pollard, C. (1990) How to take blood, *Practice Nurse*, September, 215–16.

Reed, S. (1987) Point Taken? *Nursing Times*, December 2, **83**, 48, 64–9.

Shahar, E., Wohl-Gottesman, B. & Shenkman, L. (1990) Contamination of blood cultures during venepuncture: fact or myth? *Post Graduate Medical Journal*, **66**, 1053–8.

2

Drug Administration
Susan E. Noyce and Janet Hutchinson

2.1 INTRODUCTION

The safe use of drugs requires rigorous attention to detail from the point at which the decision is made to prescribe a medicine, to the time it is taken, and its effects monitored. The process involves doctors, nurses and pharmacists each with clear responsibilities to ensure that medicines are used optimally, stored appropriately and disposed of safely.

The traditional roles and responsibilities of these three, form the basis of the guidance in this chapter. The boundaries between the professions in relation to drug usage are however becoming less distinct with nurse prescribing imminent, the deregulation of powerful prescription only medicines (POMs) to pharmacy (P) status and clarification of the doctors' terms of service regarding recommendation of over the counter (OTC) medication (Department of Health, 1994).

The roles and responsibilities of nurses involved with the administration of drugs have been re-defined in a Standards Document by the United Kingdom Central Council for Nursing, Midwifery and Health Visiting (1992). It requires the exercise of professional judgement whether the nurse is administering the medicine, assisting in its administration or overseeing the self administration of a medicine.

Authorisation for administration can be given in one of three ways:

- An instruction written by a medical practitioner on an official chart.
- In accordance with locally agreed clinical procedures.

- 'Under *exceptional* circumstances (but not for controlled drugs), an authorised nurse may accept an oral message from a doctor. This shall subsequently be confirmed in writing within a locally agreed time, not normally exceeding twenty four hours.' (Duthie, 1988)

An authorised nurse is defined as any registered nurse who satisfies the criteria to enable him or her to administer medicines without supervision i.e. a midwife or a first or second level registered nurse in the majority of circumstances. The full introduction of nurse prescribing would supersede some of these existing arrangements.

Local clinical procedures or protocols may define circumstances in which nurses or others competent to take responsibility may initiate the use of medicine. Examples include wound care or 'household remedies' for self limiting conditions. They may also provide a mechanism whereby responsibility may be delegated to nurses for drug administration which would previously have required a doctor, for example intravenous drug administration.

There are fundamental differences when medicines are administered in a domiciliary setting compared to an institutional setting. In the home, the patient or carer are active participants in the drug use process. It is important to remember that ultimately they have discretion over whether the medicine is taken at all, or is subject to accidental or deliberate variation from the intended regimen. In addition, the nurse commonly does not see the original prescription and may not be party to the advice the pharmacist gave on the use of the product.

Working from the familiar pharmaceutical adage that effective drug therapy is about giving the right drug in the right dose to the right patient at the right time, nurses need to satisfy themselves on all four of these counts. Whilst three of these parameters are readily verifiable, dosage considerations may be more problematic.

The appropriate dosage of a medicine is markedly influenced by age. Whereas children's doses tend to be clearly defined in standard texts such as the *British National Formulary* (*BNF*), far less attention is given to dosage modification required in old age. Elderly people are highly susceptible to adverse consequences of medication due to declining renal and hepatic function and alterations in the ratio of lean body mass to body fat. The distribution of drugs in the body and rate of clearance may thus be markedly affected, and the dosage of a medicine for an 80 year old may only need to be half of that prescribed for a younger adult.

2.2 MEDICINES LEGISLATION

The prescription and supply of medicines is controlled by two main statutes: the Medicines Act 1968 and the Misuse of Drugs Act 1971. The Medicines Act controls the manufacture, distribution and importation of medicines, whilst the Misuse of Drugs Act covers specifically drugs liable to abuse. These Acts, together with the Poisons Act 1972 which regulates the sale of non-medicinal poisons, effectively replace all previous legislation relating to medicines and poisons.

2.3 GUIDANCE FOR PRACTICE – DRUG ADMINISTRATION

Oral administration

Medicines given by mouth have the advantage that they may be readily self administered. They may have a wide range of formulation characteristics to promote optimal absorption and clinical effect, or to disguise unpleasant taste or irritant effects. They have the disadvantage that correct administration generally relies on the understanding or commitment of the patient, and that other substances taken concurrently may interfere with their use. Generally tablets or capsules which are swallowed disintegrate in the acid content of the stomach and then pass into the small intestine where the majority of drugs are absorbed. From there they enter the portal circulation and are transported directly to the liver which is the main site of metabolism of many drugs.

Drugs that are extensively metabolised by the liver may only reach the general circulation in relatively small concentrations. These drugs are significantly removed by this first pass through the liver and are said to undergo extensive first pass metabolism (Fig. 2.1). Drugs which are affected in this way, such as propranolol or verapamil, may need to be given in much higher doses by the oral route than if given

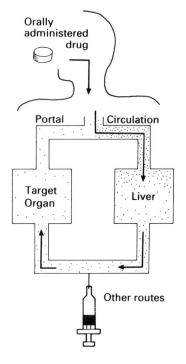

Figure 2.1 The first pass effect. For drugs with a high first pass effect administered via the stomach a large amount is metabolised before reaching the systemic circulation. Other routes bypass this effect. Source: adapted from *Basic Clinical Pharmacokinetics*, by M.E. Winter, by courtesy of Applied Therapeutics Inc.

parenterally, when the 'first pass' effect is avoided. Some drugs are so highly extracted (e.g. lignocaine) that they are ineffective by the oral route and have to be given parenterally.

The oral absorption of a medicine may be affected by the presence of food in the stomach, or inadequate fluid intake. Certain interactions between drugs will also affect absorption, for example when tetracyclines and antacids are given concurrently. Appendix 1 of the *BNF* is a valuable reference source for clinically significant interactions between drugs.

Formulation science can now target the release of a drug to achieve a range of effects. For example, if a drug is irritant to the lining of the stomach, or significantly degraded in an acid medium, an enteric coating can be applied. This enables the tablet or capsule to pass through the stomach unchanged and dissolve in the more alkaline environment of the proximal small intestine. Naturally, if given at the same time as an antacid or acid suppressant drug, this carefully formulated benefit will be lost.

Similarly, the active drug may be encapsulated into a range of coatings, designed to dissolve at different times during the transit of the medicine through the gastro-intestinal tract. Crushing or chewing these modified release preparations may negate these design features.

At the extremes of the digestive tract, medicines given buccally (between the gum and the cheek), sublingually (under the tongue), or rectally, are absorbed directly into the systemic circulation and escape first pass metabolism. High plasma concentrations may be achieved, for example 1 g metronidazole given rectally achieves peak plasma levels comparable with 500 mg given by intravenous administration (Ralph, 1983).

Oral medicines are dispensed with standardised additional labels warning patients, or health professionals administering drugs, of any particular requirements associated with their administration. These instructions are listed in Appendix 9 of the *BNF* and should be read and followed carefully to ensure optimal therapy.

Education of patients and carers

Patients or their carers should be encouraged to become active participants in their therapy. Grant (1992) has defined a set of questions (Fig. 2.2) for patients to use in eliciting adequate information from

---

20 QUESTIONS

Ask your doctor or pharmacist these questions to make sure that you are receiving the most suitable treatment, that you know what your medicines should do and that you know how to use them.

Before a prescription is written
1. Is there an alternative to treatment with medicines for my condition?
2. How can I help myself apart from taking the medicine?
3. What kind of medicine is it?
4. How will it help me?
5. How important is it to take this medicine?
6. Is this a new medicine? If so, what advantages does it have over older products?

Before the consultation ends
7. How and when should I take the medicine?
8. How can I tell if it is working?
9. For how long should I take the medicine?

10. What may happen if I do not take it?
11. What should I do if I miss a dose?
12. Is the medicine likely to have any unwanted effects? If so, how serious might they be?
13. What should I do if unwanted effects occur?
14. Will I need to see you again?
15. What will you want to know from me then?

When the prescription is dispensed
16. Can I take other medicines with it?
17. Are there any foods or drinks I should avoid?
18. Can I drive a car after taking the medicine?
19. Where should I keep it?
20. What should I do with any leftover medicine?

Figure 2.2 20 Questions to ask your doctor or pharmacist. Source: Reproduced with permission from *Which? Medicine* by Rosalind Grant, published by Consumers' Association and available from Consumers' Association, Castlemead, Gascoyne Way, Hertford SG14 1LH for £12.99 (p&p free).

the doctor or pharmacist, together with a medicines worksheet recording appropriate details of the medicines being taken. (Worksheets can be obtained free of charge from the Consumers Association.)

On 1 January 1994 new labelling requirements came into effect incorporating the requirements of EC Council Directive 92/27 on the labelling of medicinal products for human use and on package leaflets. These require the provision to the patient of detailed information about indications, correct dosage and side effects following a standard format. The information will be provided as a package leaflet or on the label if it fits, and will be phased in over a period of five years. With an increasingly well informed general public there is likely to be an increasing demand for information about medicines by patients. Interprofessional liaison with local pharmacists or the local drug information service within hospital pharmacies, will prove useful in meeting these additional demands.

Aids to compliance

Often community pharmacists have the facility to dispense medicines to meet special needs of individual patients. They may be able to produce a large type-face or braille label for the visually impaired. Bottles may be fitted with winged caps to aid opening by arthritic hands, or simply not fitted with a child resistant closure.

Alternatively, medicines may be dispensed into a compliance aid or monitored dosage system (MDS) such as the dosette which presents together all capsules or tablets to be taken at a particular time of day or day in the week. MDSs are not currently reimbursed under the NHS and may need to be purchased by the patient unless there is an alternative local arrangement (Steward, 1992).

Until July 1992 oral liquid doses were required to be dispensed as 5 ml quantities or multiples thereof. Since this date doses of less than 5 ml can be dispensed undiluted accompanied by an oral syringe. Syringes are marked in 0.5 ml divisions and are a convenient method of administering small volumes to babies and young children.

2.4 GUIDANCE FOR PRACTICE – INJECTIONS

Drugs may be delivered by injection into the skin or muscular tissues, or directly into the blood stream. The absorption, and hence effect of the medication varies with the tissue site chosen and this may be determined by the properties of the drug. For example, for an irritant drug, the deep intramuscular route or a rapid intravenous injection/infusion may be required.

Intramuscular injections

Of the local injection sites, the intramuscular route is the site of most rapid absorption owing to the high vascularity of muscular tissue (the rate is significantly reduced when a patient is in shock). The muscles most commonly used for intramuscular administration of medicine are located in the upper arm, thigh or buttock. A clear appreciation of the underlying anatomy is necessary to avoid injury to nerves or bones, or entering blood vessels.

The site of injection will be influenced by the volume and viscosity of the injection, as will the choice of needle and syringe (Table 2.1).

Some intramuscular injections are formulated as a 'depot' to release their drug over a prolonged time period, commonly weeks and sometimes longer. Although this mode of administration is attractive because it ensures compliance with the regimen (e.g. psychotropic drugs used in schizophrenia) particular problems arise if the patient experiences adverse effects. Thus great care should be exercised in the initial stages of treatment.

Subcutaneous injections

Subcutaneous injections are delivered into the tissue between the skin (epidermis) and the muscle. This route offers a variety of possible sites including the upper arm, thigh, abdomen and back. The onset of effect is usually within half an hour although the release of the drug can be modified as in the case of longer acting insulins. Where a sustained plasma level of a drug is desirable, continuous subcutaneous infusion using a syringe driver may be possible for certain drugs (see also section 7.4). This is particularly

Table 2.1 Syringe and needle sizes.

Type of injection	Size of syringe	Size of needle (gauge)
Subcutaneous	2, 2.5 or 3 ml calibrated in 0.1 ml	23, 25 or 26
Intramuscular	5 ml calibrated in 0.2 ml	20, 21, 22 or 23
Intradermal	1 ml calibrated in 0.1 ml or 0.01 ml and/or minims	25, 26 or 27
Insulin which is given subcutaneously	1 ml calibrated in units	25, 26 or 27

useful when giving opiate analgesics in the control of both acute and chronic pain and for administering insulin to selected patients with diabetes.

Where injections are regularly repeated as in the treatment of insulin dependent diabetes it is important to rotate the injection sites of successive doses to different parts of the body, to limit the formation of lumps of fatty tissue. A sketch of the site and date of administration may be kept in the patient's notes, or by the patient.

Intradermal injection

This route is mainly reserved for sensitivity testing in allergic or immune mediated conditions, e.g. the Mantoux test before BCG immunisation. The drug is delivered within the layers of the skin just below the epidermis, commonly on the inner surface of the forearm.

Few drugs are given intradermally, but some vaccines may be, and BCG must be, given via this route. In these circumstances the upper arm is the preferred site.

Education of patients and carers

Self administration of injections by patients or their carers has mainly been limited to diabetic patients or people susceptible to severe asthma or anaphylaxis. However, other therapies administered by injection are increasingly available in a home setting and nurses play the key role in encouraging and supporting patients in acquiring the technique of safe and effective self injection. This involves nurses assessing the patient's understanding, skills and ability to self administer injections, and teaching the skills necessary to inject, to monitor their own condition and to

dispose safely of injecting equipment according to locally agreed protocols. The British Diabetic Association (BDA) produces a wide range of educational literature for patients and their families. A catalogue and order form are available from the BDA.

2.5 GUIDANCE FOR PRACTICE – INTRAVENOUS INJECTIONS AND INFUSIONS

Drug administration by the intravenous route is largely unfamiliar in community based care at the present time. Nevertheless there are a growing number of intravenous (IV) therapies being provided or actively considered for home administration. Intravenous antibiotics, cytotoxics, and nutrition solutions are examples.

Intravenous drug administration in the community should be undertaken in accordance with a local IV policy which clearly defines the roles and responsibilities of nurses, doctors, pharmacists (Breckenridge, 1977) and in some instances, patients. Specialist shared care protocols should be defined for patients receiving complex 'hospital at home' therapies.

Drugs can be administered intravenously by intravenous bolus, intermittent or continuous infusion. The intravenous route should be used only when positively indicated and for the minimum period necessary.

Traditionally, intravenous drug administration has been a medical responsibility, but increasingly it is delegated to a registered general nurse who has undergone an approved course of training, and who is willing to accept responsibility for the administration of drugs intravenously. This is a voluntary extension of the nurse's role and there is no obligation on the nurse to accept this task.

There are a number of important considerations when administering a drug intravenously.

Risk of microbial or particulate contamination

Injections are presented sterile and effectively particle free. Any manipulation increases the risk of introducing contaminants directly into the blood stream of the recipient. Wherever possible therefore solutions for intravenous administration should be obtained in a form ready for administration. This may be directly from the manufacturer as in the case of potassium or lignocaine containing infusion fluids, or prepared in a controlled environment such as the aseptic suite of a hospital pharmacy department offering a CIVAS (Central IntraVenous Additive Service).

Where there is no practical alternative to drawing up and administering the drug at the point of use, full aseptic procedure should be followed. The drug should normally be administered immediately and not left in the syringe for administration at a later time.

If drugs have been added to an intravenous infusion fluid other than under sterile conditions, the number of punctures of the additive port should be minimised and a time limit of 12 hours should be applied up to completion of the infusion, due to the risk of microbial contamination. Compatibility criteria may impose a shorter limit. Infusion bags or bottles should be labelled with the date, time and drug added and the initials of the person making the addition.

Giving sets may contain minute amounts of particulate matter and should be rinsed through with the infusion solution before connecting the set to the patient.

Risk of incompatibility

The stability of any drug added to an infusion fluid or administered via the drip tubing must be checked prior to administration and should never be assumed. Appendix 6 of the *BNF* provides a table of preparations and their usual infusion method together with the infusion fluids with which they are compatible.

The risk of incompatibility increases if two or more drugs are added concurrently and this should only take place in exceptional circumstances and after

consultation with local or regional drug information (DI) centres or the medical information department of the manufacturers. A list of regional DI centres and pharmaceutical companies is given in the *BNF*.

Incompatibility may occur between added drugs, between a drug and the infusion fluid or between a drug and the infusion equipment. It may manifest as a precipitate (cloudy appearance) or change of colour, and fluids should be checked visually after any additions. The absence of these features however does not necessarily indicate compatibility as chemical changes may be entirely invisible. Degradation may be accelerated by a number of factors including light, heat, change of pH or presence of electrolytes.

Drugs normally should not be added to blood products, mannitol, or sodium bicarbonate and only specially formulated additives to intravenous lipids.

The giving set should be changed between blood products or lipids and any other fluids; if dextrose is given before blood; or crystalloid solution before lipids. Otherwise, it should normally be changed every 24 hours.

Education for patients and carers

In many instances, patients needing intravenous therapy at home become more proficient at managing their therapy than the clinicians or nurses attending them. Community nurses may therefore need to be extra vigilant to spot any problems arising or unsafe practices developing, and not equate competence with clinical understanding.

Patients on long term intravenous therapy may benefit from contact with self help groups. Home facilities should be reviewed to ensure appropriate storage of infusion solutions under controlled temperature conditions and away from inquisitive children. Disposal of clinical waste, including used sharps, should conform to the highest standards.

2.6 GUIDANCE FOR PRACTICE – OXYGEN, INHALATION THERAPY AND USE OF NEBULISERS

Oxygen

Oxygen inhaled via the lungs diffuses across the fine alveolar membrane and into the arterial blood. It is transported throughout the body to provide oxygen necessary for the metabolic processes which occur in the tissues. Carbon dioxide, the by-product of this metabolism is carried back to the lungs via the venous system and diffuses back in the opposite direction for exhalation.

This exchange of gases in the lungs is a passive process which occurs as a natural equilibration of the concentrations of gases from the oxygen rich air inhaled and the carbon dioxide rich venous supply. It relies upon a healthy alveolar lining (which brings the air and circulation into close proximity over a large surface area), a sound circulation and tissue perfusion, and appropriate triggers for respiration via the central nervous system and peripheral chemo-receptors.

Diseases of the cardiopulmonary system upset this balance resulting in a low arterial oxygen concentration (PaO_2) often associated with high carbon dioxide ($PaCO_2$). Changes in oxygen or carbon dioxide tension trigger the body's natural compensatory mechanisms. High circulating carbon dioxide (hypercapnia) acts at the level of the central nervous system to stimulate respiration, however over time this response becomes dulled in the presence of continuing hypercapnia. At this stage the main driving force for respiration is that of low circulating oxygen (hypoxemia) mediated via the peripheral chemoreceptors, situated primarily in the aortic and carotid bodies. Administration of oxygen, therefore, unless carefully moderated, can remove this second compensatory mechanism and result in marked or even fatal respiratory depression.

Oxygen forms approximately 20% of inspired air under normal conditions. Even quite small increases in oxygen concentration to 24% or 28% markedly increase the pressure of oxygen in the inspired air. This in turn improves the diffusion of oxygen into the arterial blood, correcting hypoxaemia.

High concentration oxygen may be required short term for conditions such as pneumonia, where low arterial oxygen (PaO_2) is accompanied by low or normal arterial carbon dioxide ($PaCO_2$). In these circumstances there is no risk of respiratory depression.

The concentration of oxygen and duration of administration should be the minimum required for efficacy, the same as for any other drug. Apart from the risk of hypoventilation, protracted administration at high concentrations may result in lung damage which may be irreversible (Frank & Masson, 1980; Jackson, 1985).

In a domiciliary setting the main source of oxygen is from cylinders delivered to the patient's home by community pharmacists. Local health authorities have lists of pharmacists who provide a domiciliary oxygen service. Alternatively people regularly needing in excess of 15 hours oxygen per day may be supplied with a concentrator from an approved supplier. These arrangements for domiciliary oxygen are described in Part 10 of the *Drug Tariff*.

Patients receiving oxygen are generally supplied with either a constant or variable performance mask. The constant performance masks (e.g. the Inter-surgical 010 or the Ventimask MK4) provide nearly constant concentration of 28% oxygen in air, irrespective of the oxygen flow rate or patient's breathing pattern. The variable performance masks (e.g. the Intersurgical 005, the MCMask or the Venticare) provide a concentration of oxygen which varies according to the oxygen flow rate, and the patient's breathing. Alternatively patients receiving long term oxygen may be fitted with a nasal cannula.

The administration of oxygen has a drying effect on the airways which exacerbates conditions characterised by sticky bronchial secretions. Oxygen concentrators may be supplied with a humidifier to increase the moisture content of inhaled oxygen.

Education of patients and carers

Sources of oxygen at high concentration present a fire hazard. Patients and their families or carers should be strongly advised not to smoke and no smoking signs should be displayed prominently in the vicinity of the oxygen supply. Similarly, oil or grease should not be used on oxygen equipment as it may ignite.

Electrical devices should be kept at a distance or checked carefully to ensure that they are safely wired and not liable to spark. Open fires or candles should also be avoided. Patients should be provided with a fire extinguisher and shown how to use it.

Inhalation therapy

Inhaled therapies are now the norm for asthma treatment and a wide variety of inhalation devices exist. These include the metered dose inhalers (MDIs) which are essentially a scaled down version of a nebuliser. The drug in solution is vaporised from a pressurised canister and inhaled as a fine mist. These devices are quick and convenient to use but require good co-ordination of the vaporisation and inhalation for optimal effect. The use of a spacer or volumatic attachment allows the patient more time between actuating the device and inhaling the vapour. They have the disadvantage that CFCs (chloro-fluorocarbons) are used in their manufacture, with their recognised environmental consequences. A great deal of effort is currently directed by the pharma-ceutical industry towards finding an alternative propellant.

In addition to metered dose inhalers there are a wide range of breath activated administration devices, including rotacaps and disks in a variety of pre-sentations. These have in common a means of releasing a fine powder from their containers (either by cutting a capsule or piercing a foil cover). This powder is then inhaled by a sharp intake of breath which activates the device to propel the powder along the airways. The process may be repeated as many times as necessary to empty the container of all its fine powder, and is useful for people who have difficulty co-ordinating an MDI.

Education of patients and carers

Above all patients need to be assisted to use an inhaler correctly to achieve optimal therapy and minimise side effects.

The correct use of MDIs should be checked reg-ularly no matter how long patients have used one.

All patients with asthma should be encouraged, and given adequate training, to monitor their condition with a peak flow meter, and to seek help when lung function is found to be deteriorating. Many asthma deaths are entirely preventable with this safeguard.

Patients using an inhaled corticosteroid at the same time as a bronchodilator should be advised to use the bronchodilator first. Routine use of an inhaled corti-costeroid is now recommended for all but the mildest of asthmatics and it must be used regularly to control the underlying inflammatory process.

Systemic side-effects of corticosteroid inhalers are minimal but side-effects occur locally in the throat due to larger particles of the vaporised drug being deposited rather than inhaled. These problems can be minimised by using a spacer device, in which case the larger particles will deposit inside the spacer and not the throat, and by taking a drink of water after administration.

Inhaler devices should be kept clean by rinsing in water from time to time according to the instructions enclosed with each pack.

Canisters from MDIs can be checked for emptiness by immersing in a bowl of water. The position taken up in the water indicates the level of fullness ranging from fully immersed indicating more than 70% full to 'floating on the side with the corner of the canister valve exposed to the air' indicating less than 15% full (Rickenbach & Julious, 1994).

Nebulisers

Nebulisers convert a drug in solution to a fine mist or spray to enable it to be administered by inhalation. Nebulisation is achieved by passing a gas, usually oxygen or air under pressure, through the solution and forcing it out through a narrow opening. This converts the solution to droplets, the finest of which penetrate the bronchial tree to reach the alveolar lining. This is an excellent way of getting drugs such as bronchodilators or certain antibiotics to their site of action with minimal systemic effects. The transition to a nebuliser in asthma is indicated when respiration is so impaired that the sharp intake of breath required for use of an inhaler becomes impossible.

If dilution of a nebuliser solution is necessary the usual diluent is sodium chloride 0.9% which is available on prescription as a nebuliser solution.

Education of patients and carers

Patients should be given clear written instructions for nebulised therapy and made aware of the high dosages they receive via this route and the attendant risks. Close supervision should be exercised by specialist trained nurses and in the case of asthma patients regular self monitoring of peak flow measurements encouraged. This is particularly important as people may feel better with nebulised therapy with no improvement in peak flow. Many patients are temp-ted to buy nebulisers unsupervised and this practice is to be discouraged.

Home compressors are not prescribable on FP10 (the GP prescription form), and arrangements need to be made for purchase or loan from a local hospital. Twice yearly servicing is recommended in the *BNF* for adequate maintenance.

2.7 GUIDANCE FOR PRACTICE – REGIONAL ADMINISTRATION OF DRUGS

Topical administration to skin

Drugs may be applied to the skin either for a local effect on the skin surface, or to deliver a drug via the skin for systemic effects (e.g. hormone replacement therapy, nicotine patches, glyceryl trinitrate ointment). Whichever the case it is likely that some of the drug will be absorbed through the skin (percutaneous absorption) and thus topical therapies are not devoid of systemic side effects (for example, topical non-steroidal anti-inflammatories can precipitate asthma in sensitive individuals). Systemic absorption is increased in the presence of open wounds or burns, and renal damage has resulted from the indiscriminate use of neomycin or gentamicin containing topical preparations in serious burns.

Drugs used in dermatological conditions may be presented in a number of bases either for therapeutic or cosmetic reasons. As a general rule skin penetration is best from an oily or greasy ointment base and this is certainly preferred in dry scaly skin conditions. Aqueous bases (creams) are more cosmetically acceptable on the face and are indicated for moist or weeping skin conditions, as they mix with the watery exudate and hence come into closer contact with the skin surface.

Water or alcohol based lotions may be applied to the scalp without spoiling the appearance of the hair. Alcoholic solutions evaporate leaving the concentrated drug in contact with the skin or hair.

Education of patients and carers

Whilst some topical treatments may be bland and harmless if applied liberally (e.g. emollients), others are extremely potent and can produce lasting damage to the skin surface. The development of skin atrophy and unsightly striae (darkened lines of permanent scarring) accompanied the early use of the more potent steroid creams used incautiously. Patients should be advised of the need to spread such treatments thinly avoiding the face.

It is important to recognise that different brands or formulations of the same drug product are often not equivalent as they may contain different additives to stabilise them and prevent bacterial contamination. Many of these chemicals can produce sensitivity reactions in people, particularly in the presence of skin disease, and therefore this is one of the few occasions where swapping between brands of the same product may be problematic. Generic prescribing is therefore inadvisable.

The drug itself in topical antihistamine and local anaesthetic preparations commonly provokes sensitivity reactions which may appear to be an exacerbation of the original condition. Antihistamines are better given systemically, and topical use should be discouraged.

Alcohol based lotions for application to the hair, for example for head lice, should dry naturally and not be allowed near a naked flame or hairdryer.

Topical administration to eyes, ears and nose

Eye drops
Drops are usually applied to the eye to aid diagnosis, treat infection or relieve raised intraocular pressure. Significant systemic absorption may occur, sufficient for beta blockers, for example, to produce bronchospasm if applied to a patient with asthma. It is therefore as important to understand the pharmacology of drugs administered by this route as it is with others.

Drops should be warmed to body temperature prior to administration. Patients should avoid touching the eye with the dropper to prevent cross-infection.

Ear drops
Ear drops are only indicated for conditions affecting the outer ear, e.g. inflammation (otitis externa) or removal of ear wax.

Nose drops, sprays and ointments
The nasal mucosa provides a good absorptive surface and is increasingly the site of application of potent systemic medication. Whilst Desmopressin has long been available as a nasal spray for the treatment of diabetes insipidus, more recently Buserelin, a hormonal treatment for endometriosis or prostate cancer, and calcitonin for the treatment of osteoporosis have been formulated for nasal administration. The importance of some medicines administered by this route should not therefore be underestimated.

Nose drops may be applied for the topical treatment of nasal allergy and nasal ointments for the elimination of nasal staphylococci. Their use for other infective conditions or as a decongestant is controversial. Nasal congestion is best relieved by hydration of the nasal mucosa with steam inhalation or normal saline (sodium chloride 0.9%) nose drops. There are a variety of techniques for administering nose drops depending on the required effect.

Other regional administration

Oral pastes, gels, pellets, lozenges

Medicines used for local effect in the mouth are formulated to enhance the contact time between the active drug and the oral mucosa. Patients should be encouraged to retain the drug as long as possible in contact with the affected part. Gels have an added advantage that they may be applied to the inside surfaces of dentures where these are in place.

Pessaries and vaginal creams

These are used for local effect in the vagina, primarily to combat infection or replace oestrogens in post menopausal women. They are usually supplied with an applicator and instructions for self administration. Applicators should be washed with warm soapy water if used more than once.

Suppositories and enemas

Drugs may be administered by suppository for a systemic action. Alternatively they may be used for a local effect, to assist defaecation in constipation (e.g. glycerin, bisacodyl) or to soothe inflammatory or painful conditions of the lower bowel and rectum (e.g. in Crohn's disease or haemorrhoids).

Local and systemic effects will be enhanced if the product is retained for a sufficiently long time against the natural tendency for the bowel to expel its contents. Suppositories may be administered blunt end first to aid retention. Enemas should be administered at body temperature and the patient encouraged to relax.

2.8 GUIDANCE FOR PRACTICE – SAFE AND SECURE HANDLING OF DRUGS

General principles

The control of medicines in hospitals has been the subject of three major government reports: the Aitken Report of 1958, the Annis Gillie Report of 1970 and more recently the Duthie Report of 1988. Duthie's approach was to start with the principles of safe and secure handling of medicines embodied in the three Rs – Responsibility, Record keeping, and Reconciliation. He defined these principles thus:

> 'At each stage where a medicine changes hands there shall be a clearly laid down procedure explaining:
>
> ■ *Responsibility* – where this lies, whether it may be delegated, how far it extends
> ■ *Record keeping* – what should be recorded, where, by whom and for how long records should be kept
> ■ *Reconciliation* – how often this should take place, who should do it' (Duthie, 1988)

Duthie identified the components of safe and secure handling of medicines under the headings; Procurement; Ordering; Delivery; Storage; Distribution; Dispensing and issue; Administration; and Disposal. Wherever these activities occurred there should be a recognised person with responsibility for developing appropriate systems. For an organisation with a pharmacy department this person should be the senior pharmacist.

Such a system may be determined by legislation in, for example, the case of controlled drugs, or by local or national protocols or guidelines. Duthie extended its purview from hospitals to community clinics and services, and pointed out that many aspects of its guidelines may be applied to NHS nursing homes and other community homes.

In fact the approach adopted is equally applicable in primary care settings (where most of these identified activities also occur, albeit in a more limited way). The purchase and handling of vaccines in GP surgeries, or household remedies in residential homes are specific instances where medicines are provided other than on FP10 prescription. Other innovative purchasing arrangements are being explored in the search for economy in medicine supply, and appropriate standards for handling and use must always be established.

For these situations pharmaceutical advice is available from a number of sources: pharmaceutical advisers to family health services authorities/commissioning authorities; community services pharmacists; or community (high street) pharmacists. Some community pharmacists have NHS contracts to provide advisory services to residential homes.

Controlled drugs

Particular safeguards apply to the storage and handling of 'controlled drugs' as defined in the 'Misuse of Drugs' Regulations 1985 (SI 1985 No. 2066). This classifies drugs into five schedules according to the level of control deemed necessary.

The important schedules in practice are Schedule 2 which contains the opiates and amphetamines and Schedule 3 which contains barbiturates and certain other centrally acting drugs.

Controlled drugs legislation is extensive, spanning import/export, manufacture, possession and supply, safe custody, registers and records and destruction. For nurses the important issues centre on safe custody, reconciliation and records and disposal. The supply of controlled drugs for administration in a community setting is usually through prescription for a named patient. In certain circumstances (e.g. hospices) stocks may be held and also midwives are able to obtain supplies for use in their practice on a 'midwife's supply order'.

Record keeping

There is no legal requirement to keep a record of the administration of controlled drugs dispensed for an individual patient, over and above those normally kept in the nursing notes, or on the patients record chart in a community home.

Administration from a stock of controlled drugs, e.g. by a midwife or in a hospice should, however, be recorded on the patient's drug administration record chart and entered into a controlled drug register or record book kept solely for the purpose. A separate page or section of the book should be used for each preparation. Stock reconciliation should take place on every occasion that a drug is administered and whenever stock is received or responsibility for it changes hands. Records should be retained for two years. Any medicines wasted or destroyed must be accounted for in the record book. Alterations to entries are not permissible, mistakes should be noted and a correct entry made in the book.

Safe storage

Storage requirements are defined by the Misuse of Drugs Act (Safe Storage) Regulations (SI 1973 No. 798) and apply to all nursing or residential/community homes and private hospitals. This statute sets the standards necessary for cabinets, safes or rooms in which controlled drugs are stored.

Nurses having possession of a controlled drug in the course of their practice must ensure that it is kept within a locked receptacle accessible only by themselves. Although, strictly, this does not apply when acting as the patient's representative, it remains good practice. Whilst there is no law governing the safe storage of a controlled drug supplied to a patient on a prescription, the patient should be advised whenever possible to retain the medicine out of general view, out of reach of children and preferably in a locked cupboard.

Disposal

An authorised person must witness the destruction of controlled drugs which appear in a register, that is, all but those controlled drugs which have been issued to an individual patient. Authorised persons include, police officers, Home Office inspectors, or inspectors of the Royal Pharmaceutical Society. In NHS premises the chief executive of the unit, medical advisers to health authorities or the regional pharmaceutical officer are also authorised persons. The date and quantity destroyed must be entered into the register book and signed by both parties.

A pharmacist or practitioner (medical or dental) may destroy prescribed drugs returned by a patient without making a record and without an authorised person being present.

Owing to the strict controls governing the disposal of pharmaceutical waste controlled drugs should first be denatured using a denaturing kit available from waste disposal services specialising in pharmaceutical waste.

Controlled stationery

In addition to controlled drugs any stationery which could be used to obtain drugs fraudulently should be regarded as controlled stationery and secured in a locked cupboard whenever possible. Prescription pads are particularly vulnerable and should never be left unsupervised in a visible or accessible position.

2.9 THE FUTURE

The standards defined by the UKCC provide a sound basis for professional practice (United Kingdom Central Council for Nursing, Midwifery and Health Visiting, 1992). In order to meet these standards the UKCC's 'Code of Professional Conduct' requires practitioners to recognise the personal professional accountability which they bear and to decline any duties or responsibilities unless they are able to perform them in a safe and skilled manner.

The opening up of the medicines market to greater access by patients and professionals alike increases the need for safe systems of medicines usage. The potential for patients to purchase more potent and effective remedies over the counter must be carefully considered when enquiring about current medication. Record systems need to be responsive to these developments and the potential of, for example, patient held medication records further explored.

2.10 SUMMARY

The administration of medicine requires the nurse to exercise professional judgement in accordance with locally defined clinical protocols. Responsibility may be delegated to nurses for drug adminstration which would previously have required a doctor, for example, intravenous drug administration. In the home the patient and/or carer are active participants in the administration of drugs, and they can decide to take the medicine or not. The appropriate dosage of a medicine is markedly influenced by age. Children's doses tend to be clearly defined in standard texts; far less attention is given to dosage modifications required for elderly people. Patients and their carers should be encouraged to become active participants in their own therapy. The role of the community nurse is expanding with respect to the range of drugs and other therapies available within the community.

The controls necessary for safe and effective use of medicines should not form a barrier to progress, but need to adapt and expand to meet the challenges of modern health care provision.

2.11 REFERENCES AND FURTHER READING

Aitkin, J.E. (1958) *Report of Joint Sub Committee on the Control of Dangerous Drugs and Poisons in Hospitals*, HMSO, London.

Alder Hey *Alder Hey Book of Children's Doses*, 6th edn. Pharmacy Office, Royal Liverpool Children's Hospital, Liverpool.

Breckenridge, A.M. (1977) *Report of the Working Party on the Addition of Drugs to Intravenous Fluids*, HMSO, London.

Department of Health (1994) *General Practitioners Terms of Service: Private Prescriptions*, FHSL (94) 26, HMSO, London.

Duthie, R.B. (1988) *Guidelines for the Safe and Secure Handling of Medicines; a Report to the Secretary of State for Social Services*, HMSO, London.

Frank, L. & Masson, D. (1980) Oxygen toxicity, *American Journal of Medicine*, **69**, 117–26.

Gillie, A. (1970) *Measures for Controlling Drugs on Wards*, HMSO, London.

Grant, R. (1992) *Which Medicine?* Consumer Association with Hodder & Stoughton, London.

Jackson, R.M. (1985) Pulmonary oxygen toxicity, *Chest*, **88**, 900.

Ralph, E.D. (1983) Clinical pharmacokinetics of Metronidazole, *Clinical Pharmacokinetics*, **8**, 43–62.

Rickenbach, M.A. & Julious, S.A. (1994) Assessing fullness of asthma patients aerosol inhalers, *British Journal of General Practice*, **44**, 317–18.

Royal Pharmaceutical Society *ABC: the Pharmacy Guide to Self Help Groups*. RPS, St Albans.

Sever, P. (1993) Management guidelines in essential hypertension. Report of a second working party of the British Hypertension Society, *British Medical Journal*, **306**, 983–87.

Steward, M. (1992) *Compliance Aids: a Guide for Healthcare Professionals*. Pharmacy Department, Kingsway Hospital, Derby.

United Kingdom Central Council for Nursing Midwifery and Health Visiting (1992) *Standards for the Administration of Medicines*. UKCC, London.

3

Nutrition
Simon Woods

3.1 INTRODUCTION

The primary health care team deals with many health issues related either directly or indirectly to nutrition. Poor nutrition is a factor in the aetiology of many diseases such as cancer, coronary heart disease, diabetes, specific disorders of malnutrition, such as vitamin deficiencies, and as a factor in the return to and maintenance of health. In their role as promoters of health, community nurses will be called upon to give advice on diet and the dietary management of a number of specific conditions.

3.2 THE PRINCIPLES OF NUTRITION

The science of nutrition includes knowledge of the basic groups of nutrients and the terminology of nutrition.

Energy is required for all the basic functions of metabolism:

- growth and repair of body tissues;
- maintaining body temperature;
- involuntary and voluntary muscle movement.

Energy in the form of carbohydrates, fats and proteins is obtained through the diet. The *calorie* is the basic measure of the energy value of food. A calorie is the amount of energy required to raise the temperature of one millilitre of water by one degree centigrade. One kilocalorie equals 1000 calories. This is now expressed in the equivalent standard international units (SI units) of joules (J). One calorie is equal to 4.2 kilojoules (KJ).

Most food labels give the calorific value of the food they describe. This is usually expressed in terms of a standard weight of 100 g. It is important when reading food labels to distinguish between energy per 100 g and energy per portion. Often both values are given so it is necessary to judge which value should be used to calculate the energy value of the food on the plate.

Different individuals will have different energy requirements according to their age, sex, body mass and levels of activity and will also differ according to disease and general nutritional status. Energy requirement is usually raised in the diseased and decreased in the malnourished. It is possible to measure an individual's energy requirement at complete rest – the so called basal metabolic rate (BMR). This is the amount of energy required to maintain normal function at complete rest – any form of activity will increase this demand.

The BMR has been standardised for groups of individuals according to age and weight (Department of Health, 1991a). Daily energy requirements for individuals can be calculated by using the BMR multiplied by the physical activity level (PAL). Reference values for these can be found in *Dietary Reference Values for Food, Energy and Nutrients for the United Kingdom* (Department of Health, 1991a). Energy requirements (expressed in kilocalories) for individuals can be worked out by using their weight, age, BMR and physical activity levels. Although this is only a rough guide it is accurate enough to identify broad energy intake targets.

Dietary reference values

Dietary reference value (DRV) is the general term used to cover all of the figures on nutrient values produced by the panel of the Committee on Medical Aspects of Food Policy (COMA), which was asked to report on nutrient requirements for the general population by the Chief Medical Officer (Department of Health, 1991a). Reference values for nutrients employ a number of terms and abbreviations:

- *Estimated average requirement* (EAR). The average requirement for a nutrient.
- *Reference nutrient intake* (RNI). A sufficient amount of a nutrient estimated on the highest individual requirement.
- *Lower reference nutrient intake* (LRNI). The amount of a nutrient sufficient for those with minimal needs for that nutrient, i.e. not sufficient for the average person.
- *Safe intake*. A term used where it is not possible to estimate requirements but the level is set at what is judged to be the RNI without incurring undesirable side effects.
- *Non-starch polysaccharides* (NSP). The term used in the reference guide instead of dietary fibre. NSP has been given a DRV because of the general research consensus that dietary fibre (NSP) is of benefit to health (Southgate *et al.*, 1978; Bingham *et al.*, 1979; Wenlock *et al.*, 1984).

Main groups of nutrients

Carbohydrates

Carbohydrates are a group of sugars which are derived directly from sugars or indirectly from starches and are the main source of energy in the human diet. Natural enzymes, such as pancreatic amylase, are responsible for the digestion of carbohydrates. During digestion starch is reduced to simple sugars called monosaccharides which are readily absorbed into the blood stream and used for energy. Glucose is the most important of these simple sugars. The absorption and use of glucose is under the control of the hormone insulin. Glucose which is surplus to requirements is converted to glycogen and stored as fat which can be reconverted back into glucose if required. In conditions such as those encountered under extreme endurance when diet is inadequate or in certain metabolic conditions caused by disease, the fat store may become exhausted. In these circumstances body protein may be broken down through the process of catabolism. This results in a shift in the acid balance by a build up of the acidic waste product ketones. This condition is known as ketoacidosis or ketosis.

Fats

Fats are a further major source of energy in the human diet and are presented in the form of saturated or unsaturated fats. Sources of saturated fats include meat and dairy products. Sources of unsaturated fats include plant sources, seeds and fruits. Fats are processed by the liver and a number of useful metabolites are produced including cholesterol. Cholesterol has an important role in cell structure, bile and certain hormones but is also implicated in a number of diseases such as gall stones and is found in atheromatous lesions associated with cardiovascular disease.

In addition to being used for energy fats are also a valuable source of some vitamins. Unused fat is stored within the body as adipose tissue.

Proteins

Proteins are composed of amino acids, the vital components of all cells. Some amino acids are manufactured within the body, but man requires a supply of essential amino acids as the raw material for basic metabolism and these must be obtained from the diet. Amino acids are most readily obtained from meat and dairy products, although an adequate intake of amino acids can be obtained from a vegetarian diet when a mixed and varied diet of grains and beans is taken. Enzymes in the gut reduce proteins into their component amino acids. They are then absorbed from the gut and utilised throughout the body.

Minerals and trace elements

Minerals and trace elements such as sodium, iron, potassium and zinc must be obtained from the diet. Minerals are important elements in the structure of bones, teeth and proteins. Minerals have a role in the function of many enzymes and the control of body fluids.

Water

Water comprises 60–70% of total body weight. A 65 kg man contains approximately 40 litres of water, most of which is intracellular. Water is essential for metabolic function, which will quickly be disrupted if

Table 3.1 Soluble vitamins.

Water soluble vitamins	Fat soluble vitamins
B1	A
B2	D
B6	E
B12	K
C	

water is withheld. Water requirement can be calculated on the basis of output:

$$\text{Requirement} = \text{urine output} + 500\,\text{ml insensible loss} + 100\,\text{ml faecal loss}$$

Or 30 × weight in kg.
For example, 70 kg × 30 = 2100 ml

Requirement will increase in conditions such as fever, diarrhoea and vomiting and hyperventilation.

Vitamins

Vitamins are groups of organic substances found in very small quantities in all kinds of foods. Vitamins are essential for normal nutrition and health, and although they are only required in very small quantities, deficiencies can have a serious impact on health. Vitamins are divided into two broad groups shown in Table 3.1: water soluble and fat soluble.

Deficiencies of different vitamins cause different symptoms, as shown in Table 3.2. Symptoms of vitamin deficiency may be severe. Extreme cases are

Table 3.2 Sources of vitamins and symptoms of vitamin deficiency.

Vitamin	Source	Symptoms of deficiency
A (Retinol)	Whole milk, butter and in fruit and vegetables as retinol equivalents.	Xeropthalmia or 'night blindness'.
B1 (Thiamin)	Found in most foodstuffs.	Cardiomyopathy, peripheral neuropathy. Severe deficiencies can cause beriberi.
B2 (Riboflavin)	Liver, kidney, milk, meat, cheese, eggs and moderate amounts in green vegetables.	Deficiencies are rare, but can cause pallegra.
B6 (Pyridoxine)	Meat, fish, eggs, whole cereals and some vegetables.	Anaemia.
B12 (& Folate)	Found in most animal foods.	Pernicious anaemia (B12). Megaloblastic anaemia (Folate).
C (Ascorbic acid)	Fresh fruit and vegetables.	Bleeding and healing problems, 'scurvy'.
D	Milk fats, egg yolk and fish liver oils.	Rickets, osteomalacia.
E	Vegetable oils, eggs, butter, wholemeal cereals and peas.	Deficiencies are very rare, but may result in mild haemolytic anaemia.
K	Green vegetables.	Bleeding disorders, epistaxis, ecchymoses and purpura.

rare in the UK, but can be observed in certain vulnerable groups, for example, isolated elderly people or people dependent on alcohol. For a complete list of recommended daily amounts (RDAs) of vitamins see *Dietary Reference Values for Food Energy and Nutrients for the United Kingdom* (Department of Health, 1991).

3.3 GUIDANCE FOR PRACTICE – NUTRITIONAL ASSESSMENT

Full nutritional assessment is a procedure which requires anthropometric, biochemical and haematological investigations.

Anthropometric measurements are physical measurements of body composition and development – body height and weight are simple forms of anthropometrics. Other measurements include:

- Abdominal girth
- Mid arm circumference
- Fatfold/skinfold measurements
- Mid arm muscle circumference
- Hydrodensitometry (underwater weighing).

Biochemical and haematological investigations include:

- Full blood count
- Serum albumin
- Urea and electrolytes
- Urine and serum creatinine
- Serum enzymes
- Vitamin and mineral assays.

Nutrition assessment in the community

The most useful form of nutrition assessment in the community is a combination of simple anthropometry and a detailed nutrition history. Height and weight are easily obtained and these can be used to calculate the height/weight ratio (see section on Obesity below). A nutrition history should include:

- General health history;
- Medication usage/history;
- Socioeconomic history;

- Specific diet history, e.g. 24 hour retrospective diet history or use of diet diary for one week including timing/frequency of meals;
- Assessment of general knowledge of health related aspects of diet.

The nutrition history will help to identify a number of factors:

- health related factors which may affect nutritional status;
- personal, financial or environmental factors which may affect diet;
- medications which may affect appetite or metabolism;
- eating habits, excesses or inadequacies which may affect health.

Alterations in diet and targets for weight gain/loss should be negotiated with the individual concerned taking personal circumstances into account. Serious nutritional problems must be referred to the appropriate specialist.

3.4 GUIDANCE FOR PRACTICE – NUTRITION AND ELDERLY PEOPLE

Promoting healthy lifestyles is central to the *Health of the Nation* strategy because knowledge enables individuals and families to act for themselves, to take responsibility for their health (Department of Health, 1991b). In this context the community nurse has a responsibility to ensure that patients and their carers are aware of nutritional principles.

There is no difference between the nutritional requirements of older people and those of the rest of the adult population although there are additional factors to consider. In general the over 75 age group are less active and therefore require less energy. There is also a decrease in the BMR with age (Roberts, 1987). If an increase in weight is to be avoided then a decrease in the amount of energy foods and fats is important. Increased weight can exacerbate a number of conditions common in old age, such as pulmonary disease and arthritis, and can contribute to immobility. Although a reduction in energy foods is recommended it is important that the diet remains high in overall nutritional value (Wynn & Wynn, 1993). People in this age group should be encouraged to have at least one meal per day of high nutritional value. Malnutrition can occur in the elderly population and many may be at risk of malnutrition because of a poor diet.

Specific problems for elderly people

Dental problems
Poor dental health, ill–fitting dentures or lack of dentures may reduce the ability to chew and thereby impose dietary restrictions. Referral to a dentist at the earliest opportunity is important together with advice about which foods should be included in a restricted diet.

Arthritis
Affected finger joints may hinder food preparation so advice about techniques and kitchen aids is important.

The housebound
Housebound individuals are at risk from vitamin D deficiency because of a lack of exposure to sunlight. Advice on foods rich in vitamin D, such as margarine, eggs and oily fish such as kippers and sardines, is important.

Psychosocial factors
Eating is a social occasion but many elderly people live alone and have restricted social contacts and this may result in a reduced interest in food and meal times with a reduced motivation to prepare food. Sharing meals with a friend, at a luncheon club or eating out at venues where meals are offered at a discount to senior citizens can help restore the social dimension of eating.

Financial considerations for people on a limited fixed income can have direct implications for diet. To offer advice in this context the nurse must have a practical and realistic knowledge of food value for money.

The role of the primary health care team

Advice to elderly people on diet must be practical, concrete and realistic. Simply listing general facts about healthy eating is not useful in this context. The person requesting advice should have a thorough individual assessment including:

(1) *Physical factors:*
- General health
- Mobility
- Dental condition
- Nutritional assessment, e.g. obesity, eating habits, food diary.

(2) *Psychosocial factors:*
- Assessment of social support.
- Knowledge of and attitudes towards food.
- Financial and budgeting factors.

3.5 GUIDANCE FOR PRACTICE – NUTRITION IN ILL-HEALTH

Coronary heart disease

Coronary heart disease (CHD) is the main cause of death in men under the age of 65. In the UK it accounts for approximately 170,000 deaths per annum (British Heart Foundation, 1991) and is the cause of significant morbidity directly affecting the quality of life. The diet is one factor in this condition; other important factors include:

- Smoking
- Genetic factors
- Obesity
- High blood pressure
- Diabetes
- Alcohol

There is some disagreement about the exact aetiology of CHD, in particular over the role of dietary fat, although it is generally agreed that a reduction in the fat content of the diet is beneficial to health and may reduce the risk of CHD and stroke. The UK Government has targeted CHD and stroke in its strategy for health promotion (Department of Health, 1991b), proposing a target reduction in the number of deaths from CHD and stroke in the older age group by 30%. The strategy specifically involves the reduction of saturated fat consumption for the general population by 35% (Department of Health, 1993) as a target for efforts to reduce the incidence of CHD and stroke.

Diet and CHD

CHD is associated with atherosclerosis of the coronary arteries which narrows the lumen of these vessels, therefore decreasing the blood flow to the myocardium. This is the cause of angina and increases the risk of thrombosis leading to myocardial infarction.

Narrowing of the arteries is a slow process, in most cases taking many years before the patient becomes symptomatic. Post-mortem studies have shown the presence of atherosclerotic lesions in all age groups; with an increased incidence with age. Atherosclerotic lesions are comprised of a number of elements:

■ Platelets
■ White blood cells
■ Fibrous tissue
■ Fatty material (a high percentage being cholesterol).

The connection with dietary factors can be shown by the correlation between a high animal fat intake and (a) increased serum cholesterol and (b) increased platelet aggregation, that is, the 'stickiness' of platelets and their propensity to clump together.

The role of the primary health care team

This falls into three categories:

■ Health education
■ Health promotion
■ Screening.

Many of the risk factors for CHD are avoidable which suggests a special role for health education and health promotion (Roland, 1989). The focus here is on promoting a model of a healthy lifestyle including identifying the specific dietary and diet related risk factors:

■ Smoking
■ Fat intake
■ Salt intake
■ Alcohol consumption
■ Obesity

Smoking
Although smoking is not strictly a dietary factor its role in CHD is well established. Some smokers are concerned that stopping smoking will result in a weight gain. Specific dietary advice may be useful in conjunction with a stop smoking programme.

Fat intake
This should be reduced and should include reductions in both saturated and polyunsaturated fats. This can be achieved through a number of simple measures (Department of Health, 1991a):

■ Changing from full fat to semi-skimmed or skimmed milk.
■ Changing cooking methods to grilling and roasting rather than frying and using polyunsaturated vegetable oils such as sunflower or olive oil.
■ Becoming more aware of the hidden ingredients in food by reading food labels.
■ Eating less cheese and egg – substituting low fat cheeses such as cottage cheese.
■ Eating less meat, choosing leaner cuts of meat or eating chicken (with the skin removed) or fish in preference to red meats. It is suggested that oily fish, such as mackerel, are protective against CHD.
■ Increasing dietary fibre and complex carbohydrates (Royal College of Physicians, 1980).

Salt intake
High blood pressure is a factor in CHD and stroke and there is a correlation between dietary salt and hypertension in some people. Simple measures to reduce salt intake include:

■ No added salt to food, or substitute low sodium salt such as 'LoSalt'.
■ Choosing 'no added salt' or 'low salt' tinned foods.
■ Avoiding obviously salty foods such as bacon, tinned meat and fish, smoked foods, savoury preserves and dried foods.
■ Restricting milk intake to 500 ml per day.

Alcohol consumption
There is some disagreement about the risks to health of alcohol consumption. It is generally recognised that moderate consumption has no net effect on life expectancy and may in fact be beneficial (Gronbaek *et al.*, 1994). Advice should be centred on sensible

consumption, no more than 21 units per week for men, that is, 21 half pints of normal strength beer, or glasses of wine or measures of spirits and 14 units per week for women.

Obesity

Obesity is associated with overeating and can be a risk to health. A diet high in fat, sugar and alcohol combined with low levels of exercise may exacerbate the symptoms of established disease (including CHD). There is only one cause of obesity, an imbalance in the amount of energy consumed as food and the amount of energy expended by the body. Although individuals differ in body size, musculature and skeleton size a standard body weight to height ratio can be used to define obesity: those who weigh above the standard by 10% are classed as overweight, those above by 20% can be classed as obese. Garrow (1983) has developed a grading system for obesity based on weight/height^2. For example:

$$\frac{\text{Weight} = 70\,\text{kg}}{\text{Height} = 1.8\,\text{m}^2} = 21.6$$

The Obesity Index (Table 3.3) is only a general guide and serious weight concerns should be referred for specialist assessment and advice. People who fall into the Grade I category are usually those who are simply overweight and wish to lose weight for cosmetic as much as for health reasons. Grade I obesity carries no extra mortality risk although it is a risk factor for more severe obesity which does carry increased risks to health.

Health risks due to obesity

Mechanical
- Wear on joints

- Strain on cardiovascular system
- Low exercise tolerance and increased fatigue.

Metabolic
- Glucose tolerance decreased
- Insulin sensitivity decreased
- Plasma insulin increased
- Plasma cholesterol increased

Disease
- Diabetes
- Hypertension
- Gall bladder disease
- Pulmonary disorders
- Osteoarthritis
- Hernias
- Varicose veins

Role of the primary health care team

The treatment for obesity is in theory very simple – eat less! It is only by reducing calorie intake to 500–1000 kilocalories less than the daily requirement that the body fat store will be reduced. Adhering to this restriction will reduce the weight by 0.5–1 kg per week. However, many people find restrictions or alterations to their diet very difficult to adjust to. Disciplined weight loss requires a high level of self-control and motivation. The primary health care team can offer simple advice; diet clubs can be helpful in terms of psychological support and motivation but long established habits of lifestyle are difficult to alter. More research is needed to find out the best and most appropriate ways to motivate individuals and families to change their life-styles.

Exercise

Moderate exercise combined with a calorie controlled diet is helpful in losing weight although the main benefits are gains in muscle strength, stamina and

Table 3.3 Obesity Index.

Weight/height^2	Classification
< 25	Not obese
25–29	Grade I obesity
30–40	Grade II obesity
> 40	Grade III obesity

cardiovascular fitness. Moderate exercise can be defined as a brisk walk over 30 minutes taken three times per week. Individuals who have not exercised for some time and wish to take up more vigorous forms of exercise should seek medical advice before commencing.

3.6 GUIDANCE FOR PRACTICE – NUTRITION IN WOUND HEALING

Diet is an important factor in wound healing since trauma, in the form of planned surgery or by accidental injury, causes catabolism and fluid and electrolyte imbalance and a negative nitrogen balance. The healing process requires a diet balanced in proteins, vitamins and energy to provide the raw materials for wound healing to take place (Williams, 1986). Malnourished people facing surgery have an increased incidence of post-operative mortality and morbidity from infection and delayed wound healing (Tudor & Gupta, 1992).

Nutrients important in wound healing

Protein; primary constituent of many body tissues:
■ antibodies – necessary for fighting infection;
■ collagen – fibrous tissue essential for scar formation and provides a matrix for bone repair;
■ plasma proteins – essential in maintaining fluid balance. May be lost as exudate through wounds.

Vitamin C (ascorbic acid):
■ necessary for the formation of connective tissue;
■ necessary in the formation of red blood cells;
■ maintains resistance to infection.

Zinc:
■ although deficiencies are rare, requirements are increased following surgery and trauma;
■ essential for wound healing;
■ may stimulate appetite.

Energy
■ energy requirements are increased during wound healing. Energy content of the diet in the form of carbohydrates and some fats should be increased during convalescence. Energy is required for basic metabolism and all cell function.

Role of the primary health care team

In ideal circumstances the primary health care team should be involved with the patient in the pre-operative phase when a basic nutrition assessment can be carried out and advice given about adjustments to diet. Access to all pre-operative patients is impractical but identification of high risk patients, such as elderly people and people with chronic illness, is possible.

The community nurse is most likely to be involved with patients who have been discharged home to recover post-operatively and this is increasingly the case with the expansion in day surgery case numbers. The majority of people who have undergone surgery will be discharged with an uncomplicated wound healing by primary intention. Healing will continue if a normal balanced diet is maintained. Patients at risk will include:

■ patients with wounds healing by secondary intention
■ elderly people
■ obese people
■ people with chronic illness such as patients with cancer or AIDS related diseases. (See section 3.7 for enteral and parenteral nutrition.)

Detailed knowledge of the individual case is essential for personalised care. A basic nutritional assessment should be carried out (Stotts & Whitney, 1990) noting dietary history, eating habits and preferences, and changes in diet and appetite together with relevant social factors such as support network and financial considerations. A thorough knowledge of the relative costs of different foodstuffs compared for nutritional value is important (Ministry of Agriculture, Fisheries and Food, 1993). Advice about diet should be practical and specific to the individual circumstances.

3.7 GUIDANCE FOR PRACTICE – ENTERAL AND PARENTERAL NUTRITION

Enteral nutrition

Enteral nutrition literally means nourishment taken through the gut, but the term is usually reserved to refer to liquid feed administered via a fine-bore naso-gastric tube. Long term enteral feeding can be facilitated by the introduction of either a gastrostomy or jejunostomy feeding line – a tube which enters directly into the stomach or small bowel respectively. Feeds can be introduced via the usual drip mechanism. Enteral feeds are usually commercially prepared complete feeds managed by the patient at home.

Common complications of naso-gastric feeding include:

- diarrhoea associated with bolus administration of feeds;
- fluid and electrolyte imbalance;
- vitamin deficiency;
- feelings of fullness.

Many of these complications can be avoided with careful administration and monitoring.

Parenteral nutrition

Parenteral nutrition is a method of feeding people directly into the blood stream via a specially designed venous access catheter often called a central venous catheter (CVC) or 'Hickman' line (shown in Fig. 3.1). This method was first introduced by Dudrick (Dudrick *et al.*, 1968) and has now become a routine intervention. Using this method the gastro-intestinal tract is completely bypassed. When all of the patient's nutrition is given in this way the method is called total parenteral nutrition or TPN.

TPN is most often administered to critically ill patients being cared for in hospital units such as intensive care units, bone marrow transplant units and surgical units. In this context TPN is given as a temporary support for patients incapable of maintaining normal nutrition through their diet. Some patients with chronic disorders of the bowel, such as Crohn's disease, or those who have undergone extensive bowel resection, may require long-term or permanent TPN and are required to manage this at home. Patients will not be discharged from hospital until they have received specialist training in the care and management of their CVC and TPN feeds. Training takes approximately two weeks, beginning with the management of the CVC before moving on to the management of TPN. Usually the nutrition support team will visit the patient's home and take account of the facilities available there for the management of TPN. Some minor modifications of the patient's home may be necessary to provide adequate storage space, an appropriate work surface and adequate refrigerator space.

People receiving home TPN will be closely monitored and supervised by the nutrition support team although the community nurse may be involved in other aspects of patient and family care. It is therefore important that the community nurse is familiar with the principles of TPN, the principles of the management of CVCs, and common complications. However, it must be emphasised that unless there is a policy of shared care in which the community nurse receives special training from the TPN centre the nurse would be ill advised to handle or intervene in the management of the CVC or TPN.

TPN solutions

Parenteral solutions for use in the home will usually be in the form of three-litre bags of pre-mixed

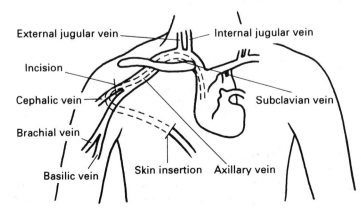

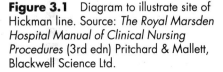

Figure 3.1 Diagram to illustrate site of Hickman line. Source: *The Royal Marsden Hospital Manual of Clinical Nursing Procedures* (3rd edn) Pritchard & Mallett, Blackwell Science Ltd.

nutrients. These bags are prepared in a special pharmacy unit, usually in a laminar airflow cabinet and under the strictest aseptic conditions. Some bags of TPN are prepared commercially and in some cases patients themselves are trained in the preparation of their own TPN.

TPN is a solution of all essential nutrients, fats and energy. The exact composition of TPN is prescribed by a doctor and adjusted according to biochemical monitoring. It includes:

- *Nitrogen sources* (amino acids).
- *Energy sources* (carbohydrates) usually in the form of dextrose (glucose) in solutions of 5, 10, 30, 40 or 50%, e.g. Vamin glucose (glucose and amino acid solutions).
- *Fat sources.* Usually 10–20% emulsions of soya-bean oil, e.g. Intralipid.
- *Electrolytes.* Sodium and potassium may be constituents of other solutions or added according to requirements.
- *Trace elements.* Added to TPN according to requirements.
- *Vitamins.* Water soluble vitamins can be added to TPN or given as oral supplements. Fat soluble vitamins may be required in long term parenteral feeding and can be added to the TPN.

Central venous catheters

The CVC is a fine bore flexible catheter made of silicone or polyurethane in single, double, or multi lumen. The CVC has been designed to provide venous access for long term use. The tip of the catheter will sit in the superior vena cava or right atrium and the route of access will normally be via the left or right subclavian vein (SCV) (see Fig. 3.1). This is a minor surgical procedure conducted under local or general anaesthetic but under conditions of strict asepsis. The patency of the catheter is maintained by a flush of saline and, or a heparin solution, e.g. hepsal, to form a heparin lock. Since the catheter provides a potential direct pathway for pathogens into the circulation a number of measures are taken to prevent catheter related sepsis:

Skin tunnel

The CVC is tunnelled under the skin so that the point of entry into the SCV and the exit site onto the surface of the skin are separated by a distance of several centimetres. Ideally the exit site should be situated away from the axilla and, in women, away from breast folds, to prevent bacterial contamination. Some thought should be given to the cosmetic aspects of the exit site but essentially the catheter must be practical and accessible by the patient.

Cuffed catheters

Modern catheters incorporate a cuff of Dacron or Teflon which fuses with healing tissue. This combination of cuff and tunnelling techniques provides a physical barrier against organisms such as *Staphylococcus epidermidis*, which may track along the catheter and cause infection. Normal bathing and showering is permissable with a CVC in place. If the skin is healed and healthy a dressing may not be required although some centres advise this as an extra precaution. Catheter related sepsis remains a major, potentially life-threatening, problem and therefore safe management of the catheter is imperative.

Principles of safe management in TPN

In most cases patients receiving TPN over the long term will be trained in the management of their catheters and will become expert in the required procedures. Most TPN centres will provide detailed training following a strict local policy on the management of CVCs.

If it is necessary to handle a CVC, hands must be washed using a chlorhexidine glauconite disinfectant such as Hibiscrub, and dried thoroughly. It is also necessary to ensure that a sterile field is created using disposable sterile gloves and towels. It is important that CVC lines are handled only in accordance with local policy and by nurses who have received specific training. In all circumstances dressing the CVC exit site, connection and disconnection from feed lines, flushing of CVCs are all procedures which can only be executed under the guidance of the local TPN centre.

Complications of CVCs

Infection.

Catheter related sepsis (CRS) may occur at any time following catheter insertion, with an increased incidence in immunosuppressed patients. There is usually a sudden onset of high fever often accompanied by rigors. It must be assumed that any TPN patient presenting with these symptoms has a CRS until proven otherwise and there must be no delay in referring such patients to the TPN centre.

Blockage of catheter:
- Turn off the infusion device and disconnect.
- Seal the catheter and telephone the local TPN centre for advice.
- Never force a flush into a blocked catheter as this may fracture the catheter or cause an embolus.

Fracture/leakage from catheter:
- Turn off the infusion device and disconnect.
- If the fracture is visible seal with a sterile waterproof dressing such as Tegaderm and contact the local TPN centre.
- If the fracture is not visible and extravasation has occurred follow the above.

Catheter falls out:
- Ask the patient to lie down.
- Apply immediate pressure to exit site for two minutes.
- Without removing the dressing apply an occlusive dressing such as Tegaderm and leave undisturbed for 24 hours. Contact local TPN centre. An occlusive dressing should be applied as there is a small risk of air embolus, (Mennim *et al.*, 1992).

3.8 SUMMARY

Nutrition is an important factor in the promotion of good health. Energy is required for the maintenance, growth and repair of body tissue, maintaining body temperature and muscle movement. The most useful form of nutrition assessment in the community is a combination of simple anthropometry and a detailed nutrition history.

Nutritional factors are implicated in a number of disease processes, for example coronary heart disease and some cancers. Further research is needed in these areas to elucidate the mechanisms involved.

Community nurses are involved on a daily basis in caring for patients with acute or chronic wounds. Given that energy requirements are increased during wound healing, diet is an important factor to explore if wound healing is to be promoted.

In recent years more seriously nutritionally compromised patients have been cared for at home. Patients are now discharged from hospital on enteral and parenteral feeding regimens. Most of these people will come into contact with a community nurse and be supervised by a nutritional support team which is hospital based. It is clearly important that community nurses who care for such patients are familiar with the principles of enteral and total parenteral nutrition.

3.9 REFERENCES AND FURTHER READING

Barker, H.M. (Ed.) (1991) *Beck's Nutrition and Dietetics for Nurses* 8th edn. Churchill Livingstone, London.

Bingham, S., Cummings, J.H., McNeil, N.I. (1979) Intake and sources of dietary fibre in the British population, *American Journal of Clinical Nutrition*, **32**; 1313–9.

British Heart Foundation (1991) The Coronary Protection Group, Statistics Database. British Heart Foundation, London.

Carter, A. and Bell, S. (1988) *Food in Focus*. John Wiley and Sons, Chichester.

Dahl, L.K. (1972) Salt and hypertension. *American Journal of Clinical Nutrition*, **25**, 231–44.

Department of Health (1991a) *Dietary Reference Values for Food, Energy and Nutrients for the United Kingdom*. HMSO, London.

Department of Health (1991b) *The Health of the Nation*, Government White Paper. HMSO, London.

Department of Health (1993) *Targeting Practice: The Contribution of Nurses, Midwives and Health Visitors*. HMSO, London.

Dudrick, S.J., Wilmore, D.W., Vars, H.M., Rhoades, J.M. (1968) Long-term parenteral nutrition with growth and development and positive nitrogen balance, *Surgery*, **64**, 134–42.

Fawcett, H. (1993) Heartfelt advice, *Nursing Times*, 7 July, **89**, 27, 36–8.

Garrow, J.S. (1981) Indices of adiposity, *Nutritional Abstracts and Reviews*, **53**, 697–708.

Gee, C.F. (1990) Nutrition and wound healing, *The Journal of Clinical Practice, Education and Management*, Sept, **4**, 18, 13–26.

Grant, A. and Todd, E. (Eds) (1982) *Enteral and Parental Nutrition: a Clinical Handbook*. Blackwell Scientific, London.

Gronbaek, M., Deis, A., Sorensen, T., Becker, U., Borch-Johnson, K., Muller, C., Schnohr, P., Jensen, G. (1994) Influence of sex, age, body mass index, and smoking on alcohol intake and mortality, *British Medical Journal*, **308**, 302–6.

Health Education Council (1983) *A discussion paper* on the nutritional guidelines for health education in Britain. Health Education Council, London.

Lee, H.A. Venkat Raman, G. (Eds) (1990) *A Handbook of Parenteral Nutrition.* Chapman and Hall, London.

Mennim, P., Coyle, C.F., Taylor, J.D. (1992) Venous air embolism associated with removal of central venous catheter, *British Medical Journal,* **305,** 18 July, 171–2.

Ministry of Agriculture, Fisheries and Food (1993) *Manual of Nutrition.* 9th edn. HMSO, London.

Neale, G. (1988) *Student Reviews: Clinical Nutrition.* Heinemann Medical Books, London.

Passmore, R. and Eastwood, M.A. (Eds) (1992) *Human Nutrition and Dietetics.* Churchill Livingstone, London.

Pender, F. (Ed) (1994) *Nutrition and Dietetics: A Practical Guide to Normal and Therapeutic Nutrition.* Campion Press Ltd, Edinburgh.

Reynolds, V. and Hay, H. (1988) Primary Prevention of Coronary Heart Disease, *Health Visitor,* April 1988, **61,** 108–109.

Roberts, A. (1987) Senior systems: nutrition and the elderly, *Nursing Times,* Aug, 12–18; **83,** 32: Systems of Life No. 152.

Roland, M.O. (1989) What is the GP's role in health education? *Journal of the Institute of Health Education,* **27,** 4, 173–7.

Royal College of Physicians (1980) *Medical Aspects of Dietary Fibre: Summary of a Report.* Pitman Medical, Tunbridge Wells.

Royal Society of Health (1987) *Diet and Health.* Royal Society of Health Publications, London.

Southgate, D.A.T. *et al.,* (1978) Dietary fibre in the British diet, *Nature,* **274,** 51–2.

Stotts, J.D. and Whitney, J.D. (1990) Nutritional intake and status of clients with open surgical wounds, *Journal of Community Health Nursing,* **7,** 2, 77–86.

Tudor, R. and Gupta, R. (1992) Factors to focus on ... wound healing, *Nursing Times,* Sept. 2–8; **88,** 36, Wound Care 62, 64, 66.

Wenlock, R.W., Buss, D.H. and Agater, I.B. (1984) New estimates of fibre in the diet of Britain *British Medical Journal,* **288,** 1873.

Whitney, E.N., Cataldo, C.B. and Rolfes, S.R. (1991) *Understanding Normal and Clinical Nutrition.* West Publishing Company, New York.

Williams, C.M. (1986) Wound healing: a nutritional perspective *The Journal of Clinical Practice, Education and Management,* July, **3,** 7, 249–51.

Wood, S. (1992) Clinical enteral nutrition, *Nursing Standard,* May 6, **6,** 33.

Wynn, M. and Wynn, A. (1993) Catering concerns ... government standards on nutrition for elderly people are inadequate, *Nursing Times,* May 19–25, **89,** 20, Ageing Matters, 61–4.

4

Manual Handling of Patients
Jane Griffiths

4.1 INTRODUCTION

Manual handling of patients in the community, or anywhere, is no longer synonymous with lifting. Lifting is absolutely the last choice when all other possibilities for transferring someone from one place or position to another have been considered. The three basic principles of patient handling are firstly, that it should be avoided unless completely necessary; secondly, if this is not possible, a full risk assessment should be carried out of all relevant factors; and thirdly, these should be acted on to reduce risk to the minimum.

Epidemiology

It is not acceptable to view back pain as an occupational hazard of nursing. Unless circumstances are exceptional, the health and safety of the nurse come first. Immense personal cost notwithstanding, a recent survey (Millar, 1992) estimated that a phenomenal 1.5 million days lost per year to the NHS, at a cost of £70 m, are attributable to back injury amongst health care workers. Community nurses appear to be at great risk of back injury, second only to nurses working in outpatients (Institute of Manpower Studies, 1993).

European Community Directive

The EC Directive L156/9–13 on manual handling came into operation on 1 January 1993 (Health and Safety Commission, 1991, see Table 4.1). Employers are no longer protected by taking 'reasonable care' as required by the Health and Safety at Work Act 1974. The only limitations to the Directives are when:

- circumstances are unusual or unforeseeable and beyond the employer's control;
- consequences are unavoidable in spite of exercising all due care.

Legal aspects

Frequently the working environment and conditions for handling patients in the community are far from ideal. A patient or carer could refuse to accommodate a hoist, for example, or the patient might be nursed in a low double bed against a wall; the immediate environment can be cluttered and the work space small. These hazards and others are compounded by the fact that community nurses often work alone.

Even in these conditions the employer is still obliged to provide as safe a working environment as possible. This might be achieved, for example, by effective discharge planning so that a double bed can be replaced by an adjustable hospital bed, or a bedroom rearranged or a hoist installed. If the bed is very low there are a number of ways of raising the height, from bed leg sleeves to replacing the castors on a divan bed with wooden legs plus castors (National Back Pain Association, 1992).

If any reasonable recommendations for improving the working conditions for staff are refused by the patient, service managers can quite reasonably withdraw services altogether (National Back Pain Association, 1992). The Health and Safety at Work Act 1974 also places responsibility for safe handling on employees, who have a duty to ensure that they do not participate in unsafe practices.

Table 4.1 Summary of EC Directive L156/9–13 on Manual Handling.

Employers have a legally enforceable duty to:

- Prevent occupational risks
- Provide information and training
- Provide the means to enable safe manual handling (through work organisation and equipment)
- Adjust these in response to changing circumstances

And implementation of these requirements should be based on:

- The avoidance of risk
- Detailed evaluation of unavoidable risk
- Addressing risks at source
- Ergonomic considerations
- Replacement of dangerous practices with non or less dangerous ones
- A coherent and comprehensive prevention policy
- Prioritising collective measures (the health & safety of all) over individual protective measures
- Appropriate instructions to staff.

Another issue unique to the community is where carers are involved in manual handling. The nurse owes a legal duty of care to carers to teach safe handling techniques and to assess their ability to perform the task.

However, as there is no employer/employee relationship between the carer and the nurse, any claim for injury by the carer would be under the law of professional negligence. As such it might be thwarted by issues such as foreseeability of the incident or incidents, expected standard of care, causation, and setting a precedent for future claims (National Back Pain Association, 1992).

Handling loads

Ergonomics is at the forefront of the new EC Directive L156/9–13. This Directive describes the application of human and physical sciences to help individuals make the most of their activities, environment and equipment (Bell, 1987; McAttamney & Hignett, 1993).

Lifting and handling should be avoided whenever possible. For example, can the person or object be left where they are or be slid, or can handling equipment be used? Can the person be encouraged to move themselves, albeit more slowly? It is important when all other options have been considered and someone requires lifting from one place or position to another, that the load is no more than 25 kg (55 lb/4 stone) for

one person in 'optimal conditions', or twice that if two people are involved in the lift (Health and Safety Executive, 1992). Most patients, therefore, are too heavy to be lifted by one person alone.

According to the National Back Pain Association (1992), the optimal conditions for lifting are:

- The feet are under the load to reduce stress on the back.
- The feet are sufficiently far apart to maintain balance at the end of the lift.
- The lifting posture is stable and the feet cannot slip.
- The nurse(s) is not fatigued (NB repetitive 'smaller' activities or stooping over a low bed for ten minutes take longer to recover from than heavier lifts with rest pauses).

Other factors to consider are:

- individual strength, which can vary tremendously;
- history of back injury;
- workspace (NB in hospital the minimum bed space should be 2.5 m by 2.9 m with no intrusion into the space (Department of Health, 1986));
- clothing. Trousers allow adequate movement for lifting and are therefore recommended.

4.2 LIFTING AND HANDLING EQUIPMENT

Hoists

There are around 40 different types of hoist available in Britain. Since Britain entered the EC this number has been increasing all the time. Hoists are frequently the method of choice when handling patients in the following situations (Tarling, 1992):

- a cramped environment (which is often the case in the home);
- when a patient is unable to weight-bear;
- when furniture in the home cannot be rearranged to create a safe handling environment;
- when a carer does not have the ability to lift safely without injury to either party.

Hoists fall into three main categories:

- Mobile hoists;
- Floor mounted hoists that are fixed in a predetermined place, such as the bathroom;
- Ceiling mounted hoists that are usually fixed to an overhead track.

Mobile hoists
The smaller models of mobile hoist are most suitable for the home. These are operated either mechanically or electrically. When considering which model is most suitable, it is worth remembering that the heavier the hoist is, the less manoeuvrable it is, particularly on carpets in the home.

Floor mounted hoists
These are often suitable in bathrooms where there is either an unsuitable environment or insufficient space to manoeuvre a mobile hoist.

Ceiling mounted hoists
These are electrically operated. They are considered to be particularly useful in the community because the patient can often operate them independently. However, as the National Back Pain Association (1992) points out, because patients are means tested before the installation of such equipment, a reluctance to pay could mean that the community nurse does not have the most suitable equipment for the task in hand.

Whichever hoist is used, it is imperative that:

- the hoist is regularly serviced to keep it in good working order;
- all users of the hoist are trained in its use. In the community where either carers are using equipment or nurses work alone or in pairs, it is recommended that their competence is re-evaluated periodically (Alderman, 1988).

Hoist slings

Hoists such as bath hoists often come with rigid chairs, but commonly in the home, the preferred attachment is the sling. When using a sling it is imperative that the sling and hoist come from the same manufacturer. Designs of sling vary, but they can be divided in to three different categories as outlined below (National Back Pain Association, 1992). When deciding on the design it is important to consider: the amount of support required; the comfort of the body position during transfer; and the needs and abilities of the carer.

Hammock or divided leg design
This can be positioned while the patient is seated. This is an important consideration. Hoists are for easing patient handling; if the patient has to be lifted on or off the sling this defeats the object and an alternative design of sling may be required.

All in one design
This design is useful where a patient is in pain and cannot comfortably be handled manually. An advantage of this design in the home is that the sling can be left in place, so that carers can use it on their own with the minimum of effort.

Two or three piece slings
These are useful for toileting a patient with the sling still in place, but run the risk of jack-knifing if incorrectly positioned. Another disadvantage is the discomfort caused by the upper band of the sling beneath the axillae, particularly in arthritic patients.

Alternatives to hoists

There may be occasions, however, when alternatives to hoists are suitable (Walters, 1988):

- Transfers are easiest when the two surfaces are of

an equal height: can the bed, chair or toilet seat be raised, for example?

■ Would a transfer board suffice? These can be used between two surfaces of differing heights.

■ Would a monkey pole, bed ladder or grab rails enable someone who is confined to bed to retain a degree of independence?

■ Are there any other alternatives in specific situations: a U shaped cushion and a suitable urinal may be of use to the wheelchair bound who would otherwise have to transfer to the toilet.

Handling belts
Handling belts
Where there is paralysis due to a stroke, or if a patient is in pain, has had a limb amputated or is wet and slippery after a bath, it can be difficult to position the hands accurately to allow a safe and comfortable lift. This is where handling belts are helpful. They allow the patient to be held firmly and close to the nurse during the lift or transfer.

Turntables
If a patient is able to stand but unable to turn safely or comfortably, and if he or she feels happy with a turntable, it can be a useful aid to transferring. This might be from a commode, for example, to a chair.

Aids for patient use

There is a variety of equipment that the patient can use either independently or with the help of the nurse. In addition to the nurse's professional obligation to remain well informed, the new EC directive L156/9–13 compels employers to keep up to date with the latest, most effective equipment (Health and Safety Commission, 1991). An invaluable source of information is the Disabled Living Foundation. Some commonly used aids are:

Transfer board or boomerang
Its shape and slippery surface enable patients to transfer from one surface to another independently. The surfaces need to be of a fairly similar height: bed or car to wheelchair, for example. The bed height should be adjusted where necessary.

Monkey pole or trapeze lift
In the community these are usually free standing and can be used with any type of bed including a divan.

Patients with relatively strong arms can use it to raise themselves off or up the bed.

Hand rails
These, when affixed to a wall by the bed, can enable a patient to sit up independently.

Hand blocks
These are used by patients to raise themselves off the mattress or up and down the bed.

Bed ladders
These can greatly assist a patient in sitting up or turning in bed with or without the help of the carer/nurse.

Leg lifters
In the community, where resources are frequently overstretched, any device which is acceptable to the patient and eliminates the need for a visit by the nursing or home care services is invaluable. The leg lifter is one example (National Back Pain Association, 1992). Patients who are unable to get into bed because they cannot lift their legs to mattress level, can place their feet on the platform of the leg lifter which, when they lie back against the pillows, will raise the legs to the level of the mattress. The National Back Pain Association (1992) suggests that a scarf or bandage can be used as a sling around the legs to lift them in to bed one at a time.

Bathing and toileting aids
The following pieces of equipment can enable either independence or safer manual handling of patients when bathing and toileting:

■ bath board
■ bath seat
■ non-slip bath mat
■ self-propelling shower or sani chair (This model has two larger wheels, unlike the traditional model with four small wheels.)
■ shower or sani chair with elevating seat

4.3 GUIDANCE FOR PRACTICE – MANUAL HANDLING OF PATIENTS

Manual handling is the last option when patients cannot be helped to move themselves, either by patience and explanation or via the use of aids, or if the use of a mechanical aid such as the hoist is inappropriate.

Posture when handling a patient

The first principle of lifting is to ensure that the lift takes place within the area between the feet (National Back Pain Association, 1992). The feet should be apart and one in front of the other: one close to the patient, the other in the direction that the lift will proceed (and end up). The knees should be relaxed or 'unlocked' at the beginning of the lift and straightened during the lift (Fig. 4.1). Lifting with straight legs throughout restricts movement and thus the safety of the lift.

Never lift at arms length because the further the load is from the body, the greater the force transmitted via the spine to the lumbo-sacral disc and surrounding muscles. Place one knee on the bed if this brings you closer to the patient. Remember to place the corresponding foot on the bed too in order to avoid twisting the spine (National Back Pain Association, 1992).

Never lift to one side: twisting when lifting leads to an increased shearing pressure on discs which have already been compressed by the force of the lift.

Head and back
The back should be straight. Leaning forward even slightly when lifting increases considerably the load on the spine. The head plays an essential role in protecting the spine. Raising the head encourages the trunk to follow and the natural lumbar curve of the spine is restored.

If lifting with one arm (as in the shoulder or Australian lift), the spine should be offset or bypassed by placing the free hand on the bed. If the patient is not in bed, the free hand should be put on a table or the lifter's knee or thigh.

Postural stress where no lifting is required can lead to cumulative strain on the back. This is particularly

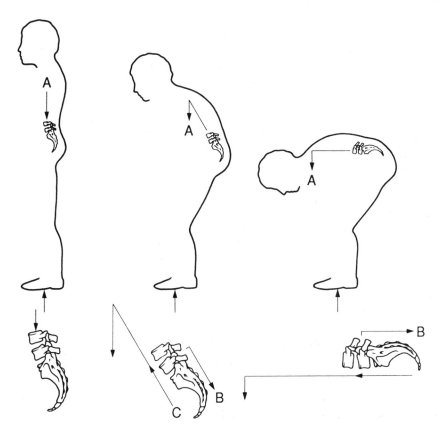

Figure 4.1 The biomechanics of lifting: (A) weight of upper part of body; (B) tension in back muscles; (C) equal and opposite reaction to compressing disc. Source: NBPA (1992) *The Guide to the Manual Handling of Patients* (3rd edn). Reproduced with permission of the publisher.

the case in the community where beds are frequently not of an adjustable height (Wilson, 1986). Leaning over a patient for a long period of time during a catheterisation or performing a lengthy dressing are examples, especially if the patient is in a low bed.

Abdomen

The word 'brace' in the aphorism 'ready, brace, lift', which it is suggested is used as a signal for lifting, refers to the recommendation of Hollis (1991) and the National Back Pain Association (1992), that muscular preparation for lifting should be achieved by flattening the lower abdomen and bracing upwards.

Moving the patient up the bed with two persons

This is a risky manoeuvre for the nurse or carer and should be avoided when patients can be left where they are using pillows or a back rest for support, or when they can be slid using the undersheet or a drawsheet with polythene beneath it.

With one exception, which is the shoulder (Australian) lift, handling slings or lifting sheets should always be used when lifting patients up the bed (National Back Pain Association, 1992). Slings allow the back to be kept straight during the lift. The use of a drawsheet for this purpose should be seen as a temporary measure.

Two sling lift

One person is at either side of the bed. If the bed is low, one leg on the bed will enable the carer/nurse to get close to the patient. One sling is positioned beneath the waist to support the rib cage, the other beneath the hip joints to support the thighs.

Shoulder lift (Fig. 4.2)

The patient weighing less than 50 kg can be assisted to a sitting position using the following procedure:

- The two nurses or nurse and carer are at either side of the bed, each with inside leg on the bed and knees at patient hip level.
- Behind the patient, with their backs facing the foot of the bed, they place their near shoulders under the axillae and press against the chest wall. The patient's arms rest on the lifters' backs.

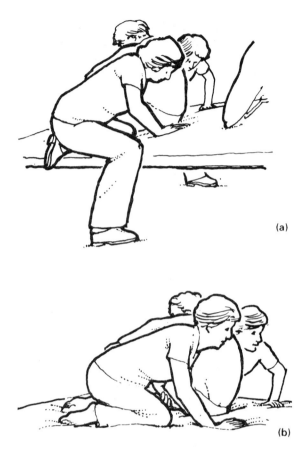

(a)

(b)

Figure 4.2   (a) Shoulder lift, (b) shoulder lift with both knees on bed. Source: NBPA (1992) *The Guide to the Manual Handling of Patients* (3rd edn). Reproduced with permission of the publisher.

- The lifters pass their hands under the thighs, close to the buttocks and grip each other firmly by the wrists or fingers. Alternatively, they may use a patient handling sling.
- The free hand is placed on the bed with the arm as a strut to offset the load at spine. Both elbows are flexed.
- At the command to lift, the head is raised, the free hand is pressed into the bed, and the elbow straightened.
- To lower the patient, the elbow and supporting leg are bent.

If the patient is in a double bed, one nurse should kneel on the bed with the outside knee slightly ahead of the inside knee. The shoulder lift should always be across short distances. This is especially the case when it is performed in less than ideal circumstances such as on a double bed.

Through arm lift (Fig. 4.3)

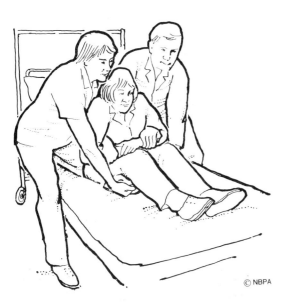

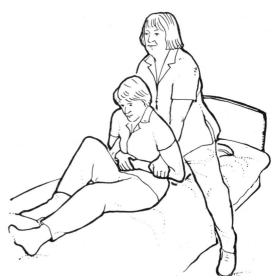

Figure 4.4 Through arm lift (with one handler). Source: NBPA (1992) *The Guide to the Manual Handling of Patients* (3rd edn). Reproduced with permission of the publisher.

Figure 4.3 Through arm lift (with two handlers). Source: NBPA (1992) *The Guide to the Manual Handling of Patients* (3rd edn). Reproduced with permission of the publisher.

- The patient is assisted to a sitting position.
- The handling sling is placed under the patient's thighs.
- The two nurses or nurse and carer face the bottom of the bed, with inside knees on the bed behind the patient.
- The inside hands feed under the patient's arm and hold the forearm firmly on top, close to the elbow.
- The handling sling is grasped with the outside hands and the patient is lifted back until the lifters are sitting on their heels.

In exceptional circumstances where the patient is able to assist and is also very light, the through arm lift can be performed singly (Fig. 4.4). In this case, the nurse is positioned directly behind the patient and grasps both of the patient's forearms.

The shoulder lift to transfer

Patients who weigh less than 50 kg can be helped to the side of the bed and transferred to another surface, perhaps a commode, using the shoulder lift. It is essential that the nurses straighten their backs before moving with the patient.

The through arm lift to transfer

Again the patient must weigh less than 50 kg. Using a draw sheet the patient is moved to the edge of the bed. If possible the taller of the two nurses (or nurse and carer) stands behind the patient and holds both the patient's forearms. The shorter nurse (or carer) holds the patient's legs, using a towel as a sling if preferred. At the command to lift, the transfer is made. If transferring to a wheelchair, the back should be let down.

Turning in bed

Where possible, patients should be encouraged to do this by themselves. Where a patient requires regular turning from nursing staff and or carers, ideally a turning bed will be available. Failing this, basic equipment such as an easislide, sheep skin or draw-sheet with polythene beneath it can be used.

Chairs, sitting, standing and transferring

Assisting someone to stand is considerably easier if the chair is of the correct dimensions, is stable and suitably firm. The height should be no more or less than will allow the feet to rest comfortably on the floor, and the depth of the seat should not be so long that the patient can slump and slide off (National Back Pain Association, 1992). A chair back that is too upright is also likely to cause slumping and sliding, as are arm rests that are too low.

One nurse can move a patient to the front of a chair prior to standing by rocking the patient from side to side while gently pulling alternate thighs forwards. To stand, the patient should lean forward and can be grasped by either the elbows or a belt or held by the axillae.

Elbow lift hold

This is useful where there is little space to manoeuvre and the nurse is tall enough to reach over and hold the elbows from behind. The nurse stands with one foot beside the patient and the other in front blocking the knees. The patient leans forward and the nurse leans over his or her back and grasps the elbows. The patient's far shoulder is 'locked' by the nurse's arm in front of it.

Handling belt

The nurse stands in the same position as for the elbow lift, but this time with the hands grasping a well fitting belt or waist band. The patient helps him or herself by simultaneously pushing down on the arm rests, or holding on to the nurse's hips or belt. The patient should never be instructed to hold the nurse around the neck.

Axillary hold

The nurse stands in the same position as for the elbow lift. This time, one hand is placed on the shoulder blade nearest to the nurse. The other hand is placed under the axilla.

The safest method to assist patients who cannot move back in a chair is to use a handling sling or belt to pull them forward and then to ease them back gently by pressing your knees against their knees.

Rocking

Rocking encourages patients to do more of the work of transferring for themselves. The theory behind rocking is that the patient is given kinetic energy which can then be utilised by the nurse (National Back Pain Association, 1992). When transferring someone from wheelchair to adjacent toilet seat, which is a particularly stressful manoeuvre for the nurse (Owen & Garg, 1991), the patient can be rocked towards the nurse a few times using the elbow hold until a rhythm is established. Then, with the patient in the forward raised position, the nurse can swing him or her round to the toilet seat.

Handling emergencies

Nurses in the community frequently work alone. Emergencies need to be dealt with in the safest possible way for both nurse and patient.

Patient trapped in the bath

Due to the less than ideal layout of most bathrooms and the size of the majority of baths, it is unlikely that the nurse will be able to stand behind the patient in the bath to apply a through arm grip to lift him or her out. In addition, this is a twisting lift in difficult circumstances, so the patient would have to be very light. The best policy is probably to keep the patient warm and call an ambulance (National Back Pain Association, 1992).

If there are two nurses and the patient weighs less than 50 kg, one nurse can stand behind the patient with one foot in the bath and the other on the floor, and the other nurse can fashion a sling from a towel to lift the patient's legs safely. The more stages the lift occurs in the better: bath seats, folded towels and inverted washing up bowls can serve this purpose.

Fallen patients

A nurse should never attempt to pick a patient up from the floor manually. Either make the patient comfortable on the floor using furniture and pillows, or use a hoist. If the patient can be helped to get up by him or herself with careful instructions from the nurse and the aid of a handling belt, this is another alternative. In these circumstances the patient should be encouraged to kneel, then half kneel with one foot flat on the floor and push him or herself up using furniture.

4.4 SUMMARY

Community nurses are frequently involved in caring for patients who require assistance with moving. The EC Directive L156/9–13 on manual handling came into operation in January 1993. Manual handling of patients in the community is no longer synonymous with lifting. Lifting is absolutely the last choice when all other possibilities for transferring someone from one place or position to another have been considered.

Frequently the working environment and conditions for handling patients in the community are far from ideal. The employer is still obliged to provide as safe a working environment as possible. Another issue unique to the community is where carers are involved in manual handling. The nurse owes a legal duty of care to the carer to teach safe handling techniques and to assess his or her ability to perform the task.

There are many lifting aids and devices. For example, there are around 40 different types of hoist available in Britain. Hoists are frequently the method of choice when handling patients who are unable to assist or when the environment is cramped.

Finally, given the prevalence of back pain amongst nurses and particularly community nurses, it is worth remembering that apart from in exceptional circumstances, the health and safety of the nurse comes first.

4.5 REFERENCES AND FURTHER READING

Alderman, C. (1988) A choice in the balance, *Nursing Standard*, 30 July, 28–30.

Bell, F. (1987) Ergonomic aspects of equipment, *International Journal of Nursing Studies*, 24, 4, 331–7.

Department of Health (1986) *Common Activity Spaces*. HMSO, London.

Health and Safety Commission (1991) *Manual Handling of Loads: Proposals for Regulation and Guidance*. Consultative Document CD34. Health and Safety Executive, London.

Health and Safety Executive (1992) *Manual Handling Operations Guidelines* HMSO, London.

Hollis, M. (1991) *Safer Lifting for Patient Care*, 3rd edn. Blackwell Scientific Publications, Oxford.

Institute of Manpower Studies [in collaboration with the Royal College of Nursing] (1993) *Back Injured Nurses: a Profile*. Royal College of Nursing, London.

McAttamney, L. & Hignett, S. (1993) A space to move in, *Nursing Times*, **89**, 18, 44–6.

Millar, B. (1992) Heavy going on the wards, *Health Service Journal*, 15 October, p. 14.

National Back Pain Association [in collaboration with the Royal College of Nursing] (1992) *The Guide to the Manual Handling of Patients*. National Back Pain Association, Middlesex.

Owen, B.D. & Garg, A. (1991) Reducing risk for back pain in nursing personnel, *American Association of Hospital Nurses Journal*, January, 39, 1, 24–32.

Tarling, C. (1992) The right equipment, *Nursing Times*, 9 December, 188, 50, 38–40.

Waters, K. (1988) Hoists, *British Medical Journal*, 16 April, 296, 1114–1117.

Wilson, M. (1986) Mind your back, *Community Outlook*, October, 11–14.

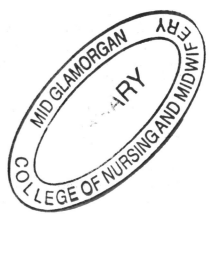

4.6 APPENDIX: HEALTH AND SAFETY EXECUTIVE MANUAL HANDLING REGULATIONS 1992 Source: *Manual Handling Operations Regulations (1992)*, Reproduced with permission of the Controller of HMSO

Manual handling of loads

EXAMPLE OF AN ASSESSMENT CHECKLIST

Note: This checklist may be copied freely. It will remind you of the main points to think about while you:

- consider the risk of injury from manual handling operations
- identify steps that can remove or reduce the risk
- decide your priorities for action.

SUMMARY OF ASSESSMENT	Overall priority for remedial action: Nil / Low / Med / High*
Operations covered by this assessment:	Remedial action to be taken: ....
....	....
....	....
Locations:	Date by which action is to be taken: ....
Personnel involved:	Date for reassessment: ....
Date of assessment:	Assessor's name: .... Signature: ....

*circle as appropriate

Section A - Preliminary:

Q1   **Do the operations involve a significant risk of injury?**   Yes / No*

       If 'Yes' go to Q2. If 'No' the assessment need go no further.

       If in doubt answer 'Yes'. You may find the guidelines in Appendix 1 helpful.

Q2   **Can the operations be avoided / mechanised / automated at reasonable cost?**   Yes / No*

       If 'No' go to Q3. If 'Yes' proceed and then check that the result is satisfactory.

Q3   **Are the operations clearly within the guidelines in Appendix 1?**   Yes / No*

       If 'No' go to Section B. If 'Yes' you may go straight to Section C if you wish.

Section C - Overall assessment of risk:

Q   **What is your overall assessment of the risk of injury?**   Insignificant / Low / Med / High*

       If not 'Insignificant' go to Section D. If 'Insignificant' the assessment need go no further.

Section D - Remedial action:

Q   **What remedial steps should be taken, in order of priority?**

       i ....

       ii ....

       iii ....

       iv ....

       v ....

And finally:

       - complete the SUMMARY above

       - compare it with your other manual handling assessments

       - decide your priorities for action

       - TAKE ACTION.................AND CHECK THAT IT HAS THE DESIRED EFFECT

Section B - More detailed assessment, where necessary:

Questions to consider: (If the answer to a question is 'Yes' place a tick against it and then consider the level of risk)	Yes	Level of risk: (Tick as appropriate) Low Med High	Possible remedial action: (Make rough notes in this column in preparation for completing Section D)

The tasks - do they involve:
- ◆ holding loads away from trunk?
- ◆ twisting?
- ◆ stooping?
- ◆ reaching upwards?
- ◆ large vertical movement?
- ◆ long carrying distances?
- ◆ strenuous pushing or pulling?
- ◆ unpredictable movement of loads?
- ◆ repetitive handling?
- ◆ insufficient rest or recovery?
- ◆ a workrate imposed by a process?

The loads - are they:
- ◆ heavy?
- ◆ bulky/unwieldy?
- ◆ difficult to grasp?
- ◆ unstable/unpredictable?
- ◆ intrinsically harmful (eg sharp/hot?)

The working environment - are there:
- ◆ constraints on posture?
- ◆ poor floors?
- ◆ variations in levels?
- ◆ hot/cold/humid conditions?
- ◆ strong air movements?
- ◆ poor lighting conditions?

Individual capability - does the job:
- ◆ require unusual capability?
- ◆ hazard those with a health problem?
- ◆ hazard those who are pregnant?
- ◆ call for special information/training?

Other factors -
Is movement or posture hindered by clothing or
personal protective equipment?

Deciding the level of risk will inevitably call for judgement. The guidelines in Appendix 1 may provide a useful yardstick.

When you have completed Section B go to Section C.

5

Tissue Viability and Wound Management
Nicky Cullum and Maureen Benbow

5.1 INTRODUCTION

Thomas (1990) defines a wound as:

'... a defect or break in the skin that results from physical, mechanical or thermal damage, or that develops as a result of the presence of an underlying medical or physiological disorder'.

Wounds are often classified as either 'acute' or 'chronic'. Acute wounds are of sudden and recent onset and include traumatic and surgical wounds and burns. Chronic wounds such as pressure sores, leg ulcers and fungating tumours are of longer duration than acute wounds; however, there is no consensus as to the point in time at which an acute wound becomes chronic.

This chapter will focus on those wounds which are most commonly encountered in the community, namely surgical wounds, pressure sores and malignant lesions. Leg ulcers are considered in detail in Chapter 6.

5.2 THE AETIOLOGY OF COMMONLY ENCOUNTERED WOUNDS

Pressure sores

Pressure sores, also known as bed sores, pressure ulcers and decubitus ulcers, occur when tissue anywhere on the body is damaged by unrelieved pressure. They usually occur over bony prominences such as the sacrum, the ischial tuberosities and heels, but will occur anywhere when the applied pressure exceeds the ability of the tissues to tolerate it.

Individuals appear to vary in their susceptibility to develop pressure sores, however there is a paucity of research to give us clear information regarding what places people at risk. It is thought that a complex interplay between intrinsic and extrinsic factors determines an individual's predisposition to pressure sore development.

Extrinsic factors are thought to include:

■ intensity and duration of applied pressure and shearing forces;
■ moisture at the skin surface.

Proposed intrinsic factors are:

■ level of mobility (Exton-Smith & Sherwin, 1961; Berlowitz & Wilking, 1989);
■ impaired nutritional intake (Berlowitz & Wilking, 1989);
■ hypoalbuminaemia (Allman et al., 1986; Cullum & Clark, 1992);
■ faecal incontinence (Allman et al., 1986);
■ fractures (Allman et al., 1986).

Pressure sores have often been ascribed to poor nursing care, however the proportion of pressure sores which are truly preventable is unclear. Nevertheless, the emphasis should always be on primary prevention, as this is certainly a realistic goal in the majority of cases.

Once present, pressure sores should be carefully recorded for documentation purposes. Sores should be measured by surface area (e.g. by tracing) and depth or volume where possible, although the latter dimension may be difficult to obtain, particularly where there is an irregularly shaped cavity with undermining. Pressure sores may be graded using a number of accepted scales. One of the most straightforward and most often used is that devised by the NPUAP (National Pressure Ulcer Advisory Panel, 1989) in the USA:

Stage I
Nonblanchable erythema of intact skin.

Stage II
Partial thickness skin loss involving epidermis and/or dermis (seen as an abrasion, blister or very shallow crater).

Stage III
Full thickness skin loss involving the subcutaneous tissue and possibly down to but not through underlying muscle (seen as a deep crater).

Stage IV
Full thickness skin loss with damage to muscle and possibly involving bone and other supporting structures.

Vigilance should be applied to the detection of stage I pressure sores, where skin is still intact. However, these may be difficult to detect in people with dark skin. Skin temperature over pressure areas may give an early indication of tissue damage, as ischaemic tissue becomes cool to touch. Unfortunately irreversible deep tissue damage may already have occurred when a stage I sore is present.

Grazes and abrasions (stage II) are probably of a different aetiology to stages III and IV. They are more likely to be due to friction as the epidermis is abraded by contact material (such as rough or wet sheets) when patients are dragged, or drag themselves up the bed.

Full thickness pressure sores occur when the deep tissue (usually directly over the bony prominence where pressure is highest) dies as a result of prolonged ischaemia. The ischaemia is caused by either shearing (horizontal forces causing tissue to be traumatised as it is dragged between bone and the support surface) or direct pressure. The first sign of an impending stage III pressure sore may be the cold, discoloured skin of a stage I sore.

Malignant wounds

Malignant wounds occur when a neoplastic lesion invades the epidermis, and may be primary cancers (such as squamous cell carcinomas), or metastases. Often a growth in the underlying tissue emerges through the skin as a fungating tumour.

Surgical wounds

The community nurse may encounter a wide range of surgical wounds, including:

- straightforward incisions which require removal of sutures or clips;
- surgical incisions which have broken down due to infection;
- lesions healing by secondary intention such as skin graft donor sites, pinch grafts or surgical cavities.

5.3 WOUND HEALING

Process of normal wound healing

Wound healing may be conveniently regarded as occurring in three phases: the inflammatory phase; the proliferative phase; and maturation and remodelling. These are described below. The description is necessarily brief and somewhat simplified; those who wish to read further are referred to Thomas (1990).

The inflammatory phase
During the inflammatory phase the body deals with the initial insult by firstly activating the clotting mechanism to arrest bleeding, and then increasing the blood supply to the injured area by dilating the blood vessels. This ensures the delivery of polymorphonucleocytes (PMNs) and macrophages to the area. PMNs and macrophages engulf and digest bacteria, and macrophages also remove any devitalised tissue and therefore constitute the body's own debridement mechanism. Macrophages also synthesise and release important growth factors which stimulate the activity of other cells such as fibroblasts – the 'factory cells' of the healing wound.

The proliferative phase

As its name suggests, this phase is concerned with rapid synthesis; of macromolecules such as collagen, and of new cells. Fibroblasts produce a collagen matrix which supports the new capillaries, which in turn are produced by endothelial cells in a process termed angiogenesis. It is this matrix of collagen and new capillaries which we term granulation tissue. Once sufficient granulation tissue has been synthesised to fill the defect, keratinocytes or epithelial cells migrate across this new tissue from the edges of the wound, until the granulation tissue is covered with new epidermis, a process known as epithelialisation.

Maturation and remodelling

This process of collagen reorganisation continues for many months after the wound has epithelialised, until the maximum tensile strength of the tissue in the area of wounding has been achieved.

Whilst this basic process remains the same, the means by which wounds heal is determined to some extent by the type of injury. Surgical incisions are said to heal by 'primary intention'; there is minimal tissue loss and wound edges are sutured together. In contrast, wounds such as pressure sores, leg ulcers, cavities and sinuses may involve the loss of large volumes of tissue which must be replaced before epithelialisation can occur. Finally some surgical wounds are healed by 'delayed primary closure', whereby a surgical wound is left open for approximately five days before suturing to allow free drainage of fluid. Delayed primary closure is also proposed to increase the strength of the healed wound (Gottrup, 1992).

Factors which influence healing

The underlying pathology

Clearly this should be corrected wherever possible; a pressure sore will not heal unless the pressure is removed, and an improvement in venous return (for example, by applying compression bandaging) will greatly assist the healing of venous ulcers.

The moisture of the wound environment

Work by George Winter in 1962, and Hinman and Maibach in 1963 indicated that experimental wounds maintained in a moist environment heal more quickly than those which form a dry scab when left exposed to the air. This is due in part to the requirement for epidermal cells to migrate across viable granulation tissue. In this context it is worth re-emphasising that the healing tissue *does not* obtain its oxygen supply from the air, nor does it require piped oxygen; the oxygen required to heal a wound is supplied by the blood supply to the wound bed, and this increases as new capillaries are formed.

Nutrition

Adequate intakes of protein, zinc and vitamin C are essential to support the protein synthesis which occurs during wound healing (Dickersin, 1993; McLaren, 1992). Sufficient energy in the form of carbohydrates is also required to support the anabolic processes.

Infection

There is a great deal of debate surrounding the effect, if any, of bacteria on wound healing (see Hutchinson, 1990), however it is important to make a distinction between colonisation and infection. Skin wounds are almost never sterile, as they are rapidly colonised by skin commensal organisms. A wound can be said to be infected only when clinical signs of infection are present, namely heat, pain, inflammation, redness and purulent exudate. More objective indicators of infection of a polymorphonucleocyte response and a tissue concentration of organisms greater than 10^5/gm have also been used (Hutchinson, 1990). Clinical infection is likely to prolong the inflammatory phase of healing and delay granulation, and should be treated with systemic, rather than topical, antibiotics as the latter increase bacterial resistance and are associated with sensitisation. Routine swabbing of wounds for culture and sensitivity (C&S) in the absence of signs of infection should be discouraged as it is costly and unlikely to yield useful information.

Devitalised tissue

It has been suggested that the presence of devitalised tissue in a wound prolongs the inflammatory phase so delaying healing, and may also predispose to infection. There is some experimental evidence to support this (Haury *et al.*, 1980).

The blood supply

A reasonable blood supply is essential to support a healing wound as it delivers blood cells, oxygen and nutrients, and removes waste products. Vascular surgery may be necessary to improve the perfusion of an ischaemic limb, and every step should be taken to avoid mechanical occlusion of blood flow, for example by a hard support surface or inappropriate compression.

Drug therapies

Few drugs, with the exception of cytotoxic drugs and corticosteroids, have been demonstrated to interfere with wound healing.

Psychosocial factors

The effects of psychosocial factors on wound healing, and the effect of having a wound on one's mental health, are very under-researched and probably underestimated. Roe *et al.* (1995) found that elderly people with chronic leg ulceration were more likely to be depressed than people of a similar age, living in the same area, who did not have a leg ulcer. The elderly with leg ulcers also worried about their ulcers, went out less often because of them, and found that they impacted greatly on many aspects of daily life. Pressure sores too can be enormously debilitating, and the reader is urged to read the moving accounts of two people with spinal injuries published elsewhere (Masham, 1994; Rogers, 1994).

The patient should be viewed as a partner in the quest both to prevent pressure sores and heal existing wounds, as without this partnership neither goal will be attainable or if achieved, enduring.

5.4 GUIDANCE FOR PRACTICE – PRESSURE SORE PREVENTION

Prevention strategies

Resources for pressure sore prevention, i.e. equipment and manpower, are limited. It is therefore vital that the patients/clients most in need have access to those resources.

Regular objective assessment is recommended to detect changes which may indicate that a review of care planning and interventions is necessary. The frequency of assessment will be decided by the nurse and may be as often as hourly in an intensive care setting or weekly in long-stay or community settings.

Little research has been carried out to validate risk assessment tools in either the hospital or community. Many risk assessment tools have been developed and are in use; some are listed as follows:

- Norton (1975)
- Waterlow (1985)
- Gosnell (1973)
- Medley (Williams, 1991)
- Lowthian (1987)
- Knoll (Abruzzese, 1985)
- Braden (Bergstrom *et al.*, 1987)
- The Walsall Calculator has been specifically designed for community use (Milward, 1993).

Criticisms of the predictive value, specificity and sensitivity of many risk calculators have been made. The reader is referred to Clark & Farrar's (1992) paper on comparing risk calculators. The aim of this prospective study was to compare the accuracy of six risk calculators (Norton, Waterlow, Lowthian, Braden, Knoll and the Nursing Practice Research Unit scale) in predicting pressure sore development. The most significant findings of this study were that there were few differences in the usefulness of the different tools in detecting patients at risk, but that the threshold scores which best discriminated between high risk and low risk were not those recommended. Importantly the study demonstrated that there was little association between risk score and the allocation of pressure-relieving equipment.

Aims and objectives of pressure sore prevention strategies

Pressure sore prevention policies/guidelines are operational across primary and secondary care in many districts in the UK. The overall aim of a policy is to reduce the incidence of pressure sores and establish best practice for the prevention and management of pressure sores.

More specific objectives are to:

- identify patients at risk at an early stage;
- plan care accordingly to reduce the likelihood of tissue breakdown
- establish research based principles of care;
- acknowledge the contribution and positive influence of the team approach;
- organise a needs-led educational programme for all health care personnel;

- monitor incidence and prevalence of pressure sores to guide equipment acquisition;
- instigate audit in order to evaluate the performance of the policy, and to identify those aspects of the service where improvements can be made.

Prevention of pressure sore formation

Basic preventive measures are often overlooked in these days of high-tech patient support systems. The ideal preventive method is early mobilisation following acute illness or injury, to reduce pressure on high risk areas of the body.

Advice should be given about the risks associated with prolonged periods of sitting. The risk of pressure sores is often overlooked as a patient is 'mobilised' into a chair. Patient and carer education and co-operation are essential elements to any pressure sore prevention strategy. It is the responsibility of the nurse to inform patients and carers in jargon-free language about the factors which influence pressure sore development and what they can do to prevent tissue breakdown. Information booklets are a useful adjunct to oral information and will reinforce what has been said (Department of Health, 1994).

Skin care

The key components of a skin care programme include:

- High standards of personal hygiene.
- Protection of skin integrity for patients at risk.
- Regular visual inspection of the patient's skin for discoloration over bony prominences.
- Encouraging of the patient/carer to take an active interest if they are able.
- Use of mild soap to cleanse the skin, after which the skin should be rinsed and gently blotted dry. The use of harsh cleansers and vigorous rubbing should be avoided.
- A barrier cream may be necessary if the skin is very dry or if the patient is incontinent.
- Regular inspection of skin areas in contact with splints, prostheses and bandages.
- It is imperative that patients do not lie or sit on reddened/discoloured skin.
- Patients should be taught methods for relieving pressure such as wheelchair hand push-ups.
- If a patient is bedbound, use active and passive

exercises to aid movement and improve muscular, vascular and skin tone.

- If the nutritional status of the patient gives cause for concern, advice from or referral to the community dietician should be sought.
- There should be a general physical assessment to exclude conditions which may contribute to tissue breakdown, e.g. diabetes, cardiovascular disease and anaemia.

Physical care

Creative, regular patient positioning can be very effective, but has the drawback of increasing the risk of back injury to nurses, and it is labour-intensive and disturbing to the patient.

Correct lifting and handling techniques are vital for the protection both of the nurse and patient. Care is needed to ensure that the fragile skin of the vulnerable patient is not damaged by being dragged along the sheet during lifting and transferring (see also Chapter 4).

The 30° tilt (Preston, 1988) is now widely used as an alternative to conventional turning, as it requires less effort for the nurse/carer, and is ergonomically more acceptable to the patient. The patient is tilted by pillows away from bony prominences and rests on softer, better-padded parts of the anatomy. The frequency of re-positioning can be reduced, allowing the longer periods of undisturbed rest necessary for recovery (Adam & Oswald, 1984).

Basic pieces of equipment can be valuable in assisting patients to move, such as:

- overhead trapezes – to encourage increased mobility in bed;
- bed-cradles – to reduce the weight of bed clothes and allow easier movement;
- carefully placed pillows – to protect bony prominences by shifting weight on to better padded areas of the body;
- foam leg troughs – to support the leg and lift the heels off the bed or foot stool.

More sophisticated pressure-redistributing and pressure-relieving beds and mattresses are available for use in the community. A district initiative for pressure sore prevention should include recognition of the fact of shorter hospital stays and the consequent early discharge of high risk patients into the care of the community nurse.

Community loans departments should be equipped with appropriate stocks, and a comprehensive range of preventive aids for beds and chairs. An organised recall system, possibly based on reported risk levels, should be in operation to ensure the movement of aids to patients in need.

Although there are few properly controlled randomised trials (Young, 1990) which have evaluated the effectiveness of pressure-relieving systems, their use is widespread and guidance on choice has been incorporated into prevention policies. Knowledge of the aetiology of pressure sores and both the patient's and carer's lifestyles provides a framework for planning care which adapts technology effectively.

Equipment choice

There is no definitive guide for the selection of support systems for patients at risk. Interface pressures of less than 32 mmHg were considered to be advisable to prevent ischaemia, but this is a simplistic view and rarely achievable. A support surface should reduce the interface pressures to a minimum; however the ideal support surface has not yet been developed. Education in the use and care of special beds and mattresses is essential both for the nurse and carer.

When selecting support systems for use in the community, the following factors must be considered:

- Is the system suitable for use in the home?
- Does the patient share a double bed?
- Is the patient/carer willing to accept a motorised system?
- Can the patient transfer in/out of bed easily?
- Is the patient able to transfer to and from a wheelchair?

Negative replies to any of these questions may preclude the use of a particular support system in the home.

Seating

Many chairbound individuals are more at risk than those who are bedbound (Gebhardt & Bliss, 1994; Nyquist & Hawthorne, 1987). The seated patient at risk of pressure sores presents a special challenge to health care personnel. Consideration of the physical environment, posture, cushion support (i.e. wheel-chair canvas, armchair base), the patient's ability to move and the length of time spent seated should be taken into account when choosing a support cushion. Choice should be made with regard to physical, functional and aesthetic factors.

Support cushions may be constructed of the following materials:

- Gel.
- Fibre-fill and polyester fibre.
- Foam
  - polyurethane chip foam;
  - visco-elastic foam;
  - composite foam.
- Air-filled sacs, including those with electrically operated alternating pressure systems as well as static systems.
- Combinations of gel/foam, gel/air, differing densities of foam.

Covers may be made from two-way stretch material, stockinette, tweed, laminated material or pile fabric. The unit cost of cushions varies considerably from approximately £22 for a fibre-fill product to over £400 for a sophisticated air-filled cushion.

Little evidence is available to support the efficacy of different cushion types nor the effect of covers on pressure distribution. To date it has not been possible to develop evidence based guidelines for the selection of appropriate cushions for individual patients.

A Department of Health evaluation of 47 cushions (out of 140 available on the market) was undertaken with respect to users'/carers' opinions, interface pressures and other factors (Tuttiett, 1990). The study provides information about the individual products, their maintenance and use.

The allocation of equipment

Equipment is usually selected on the basis of matching level of risk to the provision of appropriate aids. Such a strategy is also dependent upon equipment availability and its appropriateness for the patient. Until the level of evidence for effectiveness improves, such a strategy cannot be research based.

There are very few randomised controlled trials which compare the relative effectiveness of the different systems. The health care market has been flooded with new support systems, from foam mattresses of varying densities and fibre-fill overlays to more sophisticated systems which use air, gels or ceramic beads as the pressure-relieving medium. Young (1990) wrote to 48 manufacturers of pressure-relieving equipment to elicit the amount of objective evidence or clinical data available to support their claims of effectiveness. Of this number, 10 had only anecdotal evidence of equipment effectiveness and 24 had no evidence. Of the remaining 14, some had evidence of the efficacy of their products but only 2 had data from clinical trials which were well controlled and randomised.

The properties of different systems vary: some reduce and distribute pressure more evenly, some alternate the pressure over parts of the body and others aid turning and re-positioning. The nurse must have clear objectives in mind before any piece of equipment is utilised, if a satisfactory outcome is to be achieved.

Types of support system

Recommended for high risk patients

Air fluidised systems (e.g. Clinitron, Fluidair Plus, Paragon 5000)
Warmed air circulates through fine ceramic beads covered by a thin filter sheet, and gives the patient the impression of floating. Low interface pressures are achieved through the redistribution of pressure over a larger contact area. These systems are useful for patients with heavily exuding wounds or fluid loss from other causes, as the beads are capable of absorbing the exudate. These systems are most suitable for hospital use (see Patel *et al.*, 1993; Allman *et al.*, 1987)

Low air loss beds (Clinitron Low Flow, BioDyne II, Kinair III, Mediscus, Paragon 3500, Therapulse, Acucare)
Patients are supported on a series of air sacs, through which warmed air passes. Positioning of the patient is aided by a remotely controlled, electrically powered, adjustable bed frame (Flam, 1991; Ferrell *et al.*, 1993). Portable low air loss mattresses and overlays are also available (Alamo, Clinirest, OSA 1000, Paragon Convertible, Biomed X), but are probably more suitable for low–medium risk patients.

Although low air loss beds and air fluidised therapy have been used in patients' homes and nursing homes, there are certain disadvantages, e.g. the long-term cost, size, weight, and noise. Specialist knowledge is required to use these systems appropriately.

Alternating pressure mattresses and overlays (Pegasus Airwave, Nimbus Dynamic Flotation system)
The patient lies on a series of air-filled cells, which sequentially inflate and deflate, relieving pressure at different anatomical sites over set periods of time. Some of these systems contain a pressure sensor to detect changes in the position of the patient (Anderson *et al.*, 1982; Clark, 1991; Dunford, 1991; Exton-Smith *et al.*, 1982).

Dry flotation air mattress (Roho Pressure Cradle)
This system is a rubberised, air-filled, static mattress overlay.

Turning beds (Egerton Net Suspension Bed, Paragon bed, Egerton Turning and Tilting bed)
These work by either aiding the repositioning of the patient manually (Net Suspension Bed), or by using a motor to turn and tilt the bed system.

Recommended for medium risk patients

Alternating air mattress (Alpha X-Cell, Pegasus Bi-Wave Plus, Bubble Pad, Astec, BASE, PPS 2000, Quattro)
Electrically powered deflation and inflation of alternate rows of cells. These are either complete mattress replacements, or overlays (Bliss, 1967; Conine *et al.*, 1990).

Foam mattresses (Transfoam, Link Nurse Mattress, Softfoam, Vaperm, Cubifloat, Preventix)
Mattress replacement systems, designed to redistribute pressure over a larger contact area (Hofman *et al.*, 1994).

Water beds (Beaufort-Winchester, Guardian 1250)
Water-filled tanks which redistribute pressure over a large contact area. The patient lies on a surface cover.

Water mattresses (Ardo, Elwa, Lyco)
Water-filled overlay with foam surround, otherwise as above.

Gel mattresses (Charnwood LDC)
Combination of gel and foam replacement mattress (see Lazzara & Buschmann, 1991).

Gel pads (Action Pads, Tendercare)
Designed to dissipate pressure over a larger contact area; many different presentations.

Recommended for low-medium risk patients

Static air mattresses (First Step, Waffle Flotation System, Airtech Topper, Carelite II)
Designed to redistribute pressure over a larger contact area.

Hollow core fibre mattress overlays (Permalux, Transoft, Spenco, Permaflow, Snuggledown)
Also designed to redistribute pressure over a larger contact area.

Foam overlays (Lyopad, Modular Pro-pad, Pressure Guard).
Foam is cut in a variety of ways to enable the mattress to mould to the shape of the patient, thereby increasing the contact area (Andrews & Balai, 1988).

Bead overlay
Vapour-permeable overlay is filled with polystyrene beads so that it moulds to the shape of the patient and increases the contact area.

Bead pillows (Paraglide)
Bead-filled pillows which conform to the patient's shape (see above).

5.5 GUIDANCE FOR PRACTICE – WOUND MANAGEMENT

Objectives of wound care

Once a wound exists, our knowledge of the physiology of wound healing allows us to set the following immediate objectives for wound care:

- Maintain a moist environment without inducing maceration.
- Remove necrotic tissue and slough.
- Remove wound exudate without drying the wound.
- Prevent cross-infection.
- Maintain wound temperature.
- Protect the wound from mechanical damage.
- Minimise odour.
- Disturb the wound as little as possible.
- Manage pain effectively.
- Optimise the patient's nutritional status.

The appropriate choice of wound care products contributes greatly to the attainment of these goals. However, this choice is often not straightforward, and in the community is particularly influenced by the following factors:

Product availability
Currently only those items included in the *Drug Tariff* are prescribable by a GP, and not all dressings which are available in hospital are included in the *Drug Tariff*. This has implications for the interface between the hospital and community, and where possible patients should be discharged from hospital wearing dressings which *are* available in the community.

Research findings
It can be extremely difficult for nurses working in the community to gain access to the latest research findings. Specialist journals such as the *Journal of Tissue Viability* (published by the Tissue Viability Society which also runs twice yearly conferences and regular study days) and the *Journal of Wound Care* can help to address this deficit.

Company literature
A number of research studies have demonstrated that community nurses greatly value the information they receive from pharmaceutical industry sales representatives (Luker & Kenrick, 1992; Turner *et al.*, 1994). It should always be remembered that such information is not unbiased and is most useful for finding out how best to use a particular product; the findings of good quality research should be used to provide the least biased information about effectiveness.

Ease of use
The ease with which a particular product can be used is extremely important and should be routinely evaluated as part of studies of effectiveness.

Personal and patients' preferences
The personal preferences of health care professionals for particular products should not override the evidence if one treatment strategy has been shown to be more effective than another. Similarly patients should be placed in a position to make an informed choice about their treatment.

Wound care in the community

A number of factors dictate that wound care in the community is influenced by somewhat different considerations to that delivered in hospital. Aside from the problems of product availability, community nurses usually have reduced or no access to wound care specialist nurses who are often available in the hospital to give expert advice on the care of particularly difficult or unusual wounds, or the use of new products. Patients nursed in the community may require less intensive nursing care than those in hospital, and therefore there is not the same opportunity to monitor a patient or their wound so closely, or to redress the wound so frequently. The environment in which a patient is cared for is probably an important factor in both pressure sore prevention and wound care, and whilst this is carefully controlled in hospital, this is often not the case in the patient's own home where the circumstances may not be ideal. All these factors must be taken into account when planning a wound care package for the patient in the community.

Wound assessment

The assessment of a patient with a wound should include the following:

Threat to the immediate wellbeing of the patient
Signs of severe haemorrhage, or dehiscence of an abdominal wound, for example, will necessitate the delivery of first aid and transfer of the patient to hospital.

Careful consideration of the cause of the wound
There may be the opportunity to remove or reverse this cause as part of treatment. Pressure must be relieved from pressure sores, and venous hypertension must be reversed by the application of compression to patients with venous ulcers.

The presence of dirt, slough, necrotic tissue
Acute wounds obviously contaminated by dirt should be carefully and gently cleaned either by irrigation or swabbing, using warmed saline or povidone-iodine. Slough and necrotic tissue should be removed from any wound as they delay healing by prolonging the inflammatory phase. Mechanical or surgical removal of necrotic tissue is the most expedient, but must be left to those who are competent to execute it. Modern

wound management materials such as hydrogels and hydrocolloids promote desloughing and debridement by maintaining a moist wound environment and promoting autolysis.

The amount and appearance of wound exudate
The amount of exudate produced by a wound reduces as it heals, and exudate may change in character and volume in the presence of infection. The volume of exudate is an important factor to be considered when choosing a dressing. Some wound dressings cannot cope with a high volume of exudate, whereas hydrocolloids, foams and alginates are able to cope with a greater range of exudate volume.

A moist wound environment promotes epithelialisation, and therefore a dry wound bed requires the application of a moisture-retaining dressing.

Purulent, malodorous exudate heralds the presence of clinical infection, the treatment for which is systemic, not topical, antibiotics.

The appearance and condition of the surrounding skin
The skin surrounding a wound is red and inflamed in the presence of infection, or if the patient is allergic to one of the wound treatments. If the surrounding skin is very friable, tape should not be applied. Dry, scaly skin (which often surrounds venous ulcers, for example) is best hydrated using a simple emollient such as white soft paraffin.

The presence of clinical infection
This is heralded by inflammation and redness, pain, purulent exudate and odour. Infection should be treated by systemic rather than topical antibiotics.

The size of the wound, including depth
Measurement of the size and shape of the wound is essential for choosing the correct size dressing, and for monitoring healing. Some manufacturers specify the size of the margin to be allowed between the edge of the wound and the edge of the dressing.

The stage of healing of the wound
Wounds which are granulating or epithelialising require the maintenance of a moist environment in order to facilitate the process of healing. The major determinant of dressing choice is often the level of exudate produced and whether a cavity is present or not. As a general rule, the presence of infection will necessitate more frequent dressing changes.

The extent of pain a patient is experiencing
The precise cause of wound-related pain should be

ascertained as carefully as possible. Causes include infection, a dry wound bed, and trauma. The application and removal of dressings should not cause pain. If they do, the choice of dressing, or the dressing technique, should be reviewed.

The anatomical site of the wound
The wound site has implications for the choice of dressing. Areas subjected to repeated loading and movement (e.g. the sacrum) will require self-adhesive, sturdy dressings.

Blood supply
The blood supply to the area of the wound must be sufficient to support the healing process, and can be assessed in part by observation of the colour and temperature of the surrounding tissue.

Malnourishment
Does the patient appear frankly malnourished? Patients who are should be referred to the community dietician.

Choosing a dressing

Modern wound management products are numerous and possess different properties and characteristics. It is important to note that few comparative data are available to guide the choice of different products for use in specific situations.

The following is a rough guide to product selection based on personal experience of the products in use. Accurate interpretation of wound assessment data and knowledge of the properties of the materials should aid selection. The guide is based on wound depth:

Grade II wounds (partial-thickness wounds)
- low-adherent dressings (e.g. NA Dressing – Johnson & Johnson; Tricotex – Smith & Nephew);
- vapour-permeable film dressings (e.g. Opsite – Smith & Nephew; Tegaderm – 3M);
- hydrocolloid dressings (e.g. Granuflex – Convatec; Comfeel – Coloplast);
- hydrogel dressings (e.g. Intrasite Gel – Smith & Nephew).

Grade III wounds (full-thickness wounds, cavities)
- hydrocolloid dressings +/– hydrocolloid pastes, beads or granules;
- alginates (including alginate rope) (e.g. Kaltostat – Britcair);

- foam dressings (sheets and cavity fillers) (e.g. Lyofoam – Seton; Allevyn – Smith & Nephew);
- hydrogels.

Grade IV wounds (full-thickness wounds and cavities with undermining and/or involvement of muscle, bone, tendon)
As for cavity wounds, except beware of cavity fillers which may disintegrate and shed particles.

The clinical appearance of the wound and the volume of exudate will also influence dressing selection:

Black, necrotic wounds
(surgical debridement)
- Hydrogels
- Hydrocolloids
- Enzymatic preparations (e.g. Varidase – Lederle)

Sloughy wounds
- Hydrocolloids
- Alginates
- Polysaccharide paste or beads
- Sugar paste

Infected wounds
(systemic antibiotics)
- Alginate sheets/rope
- Iodine-containing paste/beads (e.g. Iodosorb – Perstorp Pharma)
- Sugar paste

Granulating wounds
- Hydrocolloids and/or pastes/granules
- Hydrogels
- Alginates
- Foam dressings (sheets and cavity-fillers)

Epithelialising wounds
- Vapour-permeable film dressings
- Hydrocolloids
- Low-adherent dressings
- Sheet foam dressings

Malodorous and fungating lesions
- Metronidazole mixed with a hydrogel
- Activated charcoal dressings

The volume of exudate produced by a wound is also an important factor in dressing choice. Foam and alginate dressings have a large absorptive capacity, and are useful for medium–highly exuding wounds. By contrast, vapour-permeable films and hydrogels are useful for wounds with low–medium exudate volume.

Deviations from normal healing

Any deviation from the normal healing process is a sign that healing is either not taking place or that the process is being interfered with at a local level by infection or by an underlying disease.

Some of the more commonly encountered problems include:

- Haemorrhage and haematoma
- Wound infection
- Wound dehiscence
- Delayed healing/non-healing
- Sinuses and fistulae.

Haemorrhage and haematoma

Haemorrhage leads to a reduced peripheral blood supply, thereby reducing oxygen availability and potentially delaying wound healing.

Haemorrhage may be rapid or insidious; it may be marked by overt bleeding onto a dressing or slow oozing into the tissues surrounding a wound. The patient may be clinically shocked in the first instance, and require general emergency support measures and return to the operating theatre for exploration.

Secondary haemorrhage may be due to erosion of a blood vessel secondary to infection, and may lead to the formation of a haematoma at the wound site.

A haematoma is a collection of blood in the tissues, and is problematic as it provides a growth medium for bacteria, causes tension in the wound, and may lead to fibrosis and the formation of excessive scar tissue.

Wound infection

Skin wounds are commonly colonised by bacteria, i.e. non-pathogenic streptococci, staphylococci and pseudomonas. Infection is caused by invasion of organisms into viable tissue resulting in the clinical signs of increased pain, swelling, redness, pus, raised temperature at the wound site, tachycardia and pyrexia. Infection in a wound delays healing, causes further tissue damage and increases scar tissue.

Treatment of wound infection includes:

- facilitation of drainage;
- administration of systemic antibiotics;
- administration of analgesia if necessary;
- removal of pus and debris;
- management of odour;
- appropriate wound management;

- general physical and psychological support;
- documentation of all observations and actions taken.

The reader is referred to Dealey (1994) for a more comprehensive review of the management of infected wounds.

Wound dehiscence

Wound dehiscence is the breakdown of all or part of a wound, and may or may not be associated with infection, abdominal distension and pulmonary complications. A burst abdominal wound may reveal bowel and is very distressing for the patient and family.

To treat wound dehiscence the wound should be covered with sterile swabs soaked in sterile saline warmed to body temperature. The patient will need reassurance, and will probably attend theatre for a surgical repair of the wound. Healing by secondary intention may be considered if evisceration has not occurred, in which case correct long-term wound management will be necessary.

Delayed and non-healing wounds

Delayed and non-healing wounds may be caused by:

- chronic infection;
- lack of identification and management of the underlying cause of the wound;
- malignant disease;
- inaccurate wound assessment and inappropriate treatment choices;
- ischaemia;
- long term steroid administration;
- malnutrition (McLaren, 1992), vitamin deficiency (A, C, D, E, K), zinc deficiency;
- size and anatomical location of the wound;
- cytotoxic agents;
- the presence of foreign bodies;
- the presence of devitalised tissue;
- patient interference.

The management of delayed or non healing wounds requires the community nurse to:

- investigate reasons for non or delayed healing, reverse causative factors and minimise any deficiency;
- obtain patient co-operation;

- avoid the use of caustic cleansing agents;
- remove devitalised tissue (either surgically or with appropriate wound management materials);
- give advice tailored to individuals and their unique circumstances;
- construct a care plan which reflects patient needs and evaluate it regularly.

Sinuses and fistulae

A sinus is a blind tract which opens onto an epithelial surface (Davis *et al.*, 1992). Sinuses may originate from an abscess or deep foreign body, e.g. a suture. Discharge may be frank pus or sero-sanguinous fluid. The most effective treatment is surgical excision to remove the causative factor and laying open of the area to allow healing by secondary intention.

A fistula is an abnormal track connecting one viscus with another, or one viscus to the skin (Dealey, 1994).

Fistulae may be caused by:

- congenital factors;
- disease – Crohn's disease;
- trauma – stabbing injury;
- iatrogenic - following surgery;
- the planned formation of a stoma.

If a fistula is unplanned, its origin should be identified where possible by analysis of the amount, colour, and pH of the exudate, and the effect it has on surrounding skin.

In both sinuses and fistulae, the full extent of the wound cannot be seen readily, therefore special X-ray techniques may be used.

The principal nursing responsibilities when caring for a patient with a sinus or fistula include:

- care of the surrounding skin;
- giving general explanation and support to the patient and family;
- the collection and measurement of all leaking fluid;
- observation of nutritional status and fluid intake;
- local wound management to encourage healing from the base of the wound.

Many variations are available in the form of composite dressings, e.g. alginate island dressings, but at present many are not available on the the *Drug Tariff*.

Fungating wounds

The occurrence of such lesions can be a source of acute distress for patients and their families. The lesions may be painful, malodorous, bleed easily, produce large volumes of exudate and be cosmetically unacceptable. The aim of patient management is to agree a care plan which meets the needs of the individual physically, socially and psychologically. There are no definitive treatments; much is left to trial and error.

The objectives of the care plan include:

- pain control;
- sensitive patient assessment;
- accurate wound assessment;
- effective management of the exudate;
- odour containment;
- infection prevention/management;
- prevention/control of bleeding in fragile tissue;
- dressing selection which is acceptable to the patient;
- care of surrounding skin, particularly following radiation;
- assistance for the patient in coping with the problem.

5.6 SUMMARY

In the context of pressure sore management a local district-wide policy is highly recommended in order to standardise and promote best practice.

It is important for all community nurses to have a good working knowledge of the physiology and pathophysiology of wounds and wound healing. This knowledge is the basis for an accurate assessment of patients with wounds and underpins the delivery of appropriate wound management strategies, including the choice of dressing.

Good quality research is lacking to guide the choice of products for use in specific situations. Until this deficit in knowledge is overcome, wound care will remain largely pragmatic. Whilst there is a need for cost-containment in community prescribing, it is clear that the lack of availability in the community of certain types and sizes of product militates against the provision of the most appropriate care for certain patients. Finally, it is clear that good nursing care and best wound management practice can make a positive difference to wound healing rates and patients' quality of life.

5.7 REFERENCES AND FURTHER READING

Abruzzese, R.S. (1985) Early assessment and prevention of pressure sores. In *Chronic Ulcers of the Skin* (Ed. by B.Y. Lee), 1-19. McGraw-Hill Book Company, New York.

Adam, K. & Oswald, I. (1984) Sleep helps healing, *British Medical Journal*, **289**, 1400–1401.

Allman, R.M., Laprade, C.A., Noel, L.B., Walker, J.M., Moorer, C.A., Dear, M.R. and Smith, C.R. (1986) Pressure sores amongst hospitalized patients, *Annals of Internal Medicine*, **105**, 337–42.

Allman, R.M, Walker, J.M., Hart, M.K., Laprade, C.A., Noel, L.B. and Smith, C.R. (1987) Air fluidized beds or conventional therapy for pressure sores, *Annals of Internal Medicine*, **107**, 641–8.

Anderson, K.E., Jensen, O., Kvorning, S.A. and Bach, E. (1982) Decubitus prophylaxis: a prospective trial on the efficiency of alternating pressure air mattresses and water-filled mattresses, *Acta Dermatovener* (Stockholm) **63**, 227–30.

Andrews, J. and Balai, R. (1988) The prevention and treatment of pressure sores by use of pressure distributing mattresses, *Care Science and Practice*, **7**, 72–6.

Bergstrom, N., Braden, B. and Laquazza, A. (1987) The Braden scale for predicting pressure sore risk, *Nursing Research*, **36**, 205–210.

Berlowitz, C.R. and Wilking, V.B. (1989) Risk factors for pressure sores, *Journal of American Geriatric Society*, **37**, 1043–1050.

Bliss, M. (1967) Preventing pressure sores in hospital: controlled trial of a large celled ripple mattress. *British Medical Journal*, **1**, 394–7.

Clark, M. (1991) Comparison of the pressure re-distributing attributes of a selection of bed mattresses used to prevent pressure sores, *Journal of Tissue Viability*, **1**, 65–7.

Clark, M. and Farrar, S. (1992) Comparison of pressure sore risk calculators. In *Proceedings of the 1st Conference on Advances in Wound Management* (Ed. by K.G. Harding, D.L. Leaper, T.D. Turner), 158–62. Macmillan Magazines Ltd, London.

Conine, T., Daechsel, D. and Lau, M. (1990) The role of alternating air and silicore overlays in preventing decubitus ulcers, *International Journal of Rehabilitation Research*, **13**, 57–65.

Cullum, N.A. and Clark, M. (1992) Intrinsic factors associated with pressure sores in elderly people, *Journal of Advanced Nursing*, **17**, 427–31.

Davis, M.H., Dunkley, P., Harden, R. M., Harding, K., Laidlaw, J.M., Morris, A.M., Wood, R.A.B. (1992) *The Wound Programme*. Centre for Medical Education, Dundee.

Dealey, C. (1994) *The Care of Wounds*. Blackwell Scientific Publications, Oxford.

Department of Health (1994) *Your Guide to Pressure Sores*. Department of Health, London.

Dickersin, J.W.T. (1993) Ascorbic acid, zinc and wound healing, *Journal of Wound Care*, **2**, 350–3.

Dunford, C. (1991) A clinical evaluation of the Nimbus, *Journal of Tissue Viability*, **1**, 75–8.

Exton–Smith, A.N. and Sherwin, R.W (1961) The prevention of pressure sores: significance of spontaneous bodily movements, *The Lancet*, **ii**, 1124–7.

Exton-Smith, A.N., Overstall, P.W., Wedgewood, J. and Wallace, G. (1982) Use of the 'Airwave system' to prevent pressure sores, *The Lancet*, **i**, 1288–90.

Ferrell, B.A., Osterweil, D. and Christenson, P. (1993) A randomised trial of low air loss beds for treatment of pressure ulcers, *Journal of the American Medical Association*, **269**, 494–7.

Flam, E. (1991) A new risk factor analysis, *Journal of Extended Patient Care Management*, **1**, 28.

Gebhardt, K. and Bliss, M.R. (1994) Preventing pressure sores in orthopaedic patients – is prolonged chair nursing detrimental? *Journal of Tissue Viability*, **4**, 51–4.

Gosnell, D.J. (1973) An assessment tool to identify pressure sores, *Nursing Research*, **22**, 55–9.

Gottrup, F. (1992) Advances in the biology of wound healing. In *Proceedings of the 1st European Conference on Advances in Wound Management* (Ed. by K.G. Harding, D.L. Leaper, T.D. Turner), 7–10. Macmillan Magazines Ltd, London.

Haury, B., Rodeheaver, G., Vensko, J., Edgerton, M.T. and Edlich, R.F. (1980) Debridement: an essential component of traumatic wound care. *Wound Healing and Wound Infection: Theory and Surgical Practice* (Ed. by T.K. Hunt), 229–41 Apple-Century-Crofts, New York.

Hinman, C.D. and Maibach, H. (1963) Effect of air exposure and occlusion on experimental human skin wounds, *Nature*, **200**, 377–8.

Hofman, A., Geelkerken, R., Wille, J., Hamming, J., Hermans, J. and Breslau, P. (1994) Pressure sores and pressure decreasing mattresses: controlled clinical trial, *The Lancet*, **343**, 568–71.

Hutchinson, J.J. (1990) The rate of clinical infection in occluded wounds. In *International Forum on Wound Microbiology*. (Ed. by J.W. Alexander, P.D. Thomson, J.J. Hutchinson), 27–34. Excerpta Medica, Princeton.

Lazzara, D. and Buschmann, M. (1991) Prevention of pressure sores in elderly nursing home residents: are special support surfaces the answer? *Decubitus*, **4**, 42–8.

Lowthian, P.T. (1987) The practical assessment of pressure sore risk, *Care Science & Practice*, **5**, 3–7.

Luker, K.A. and Kenrick, M. (1992) An exploratory study of the sources of influence on the clinical decisions of community nurses. *Journal of Advanced Nursing*, **17**, 457–466.

Masham of Ilton, Baroness (1994) Healing – the patient's perspective. In *Proceedings of the 3rd Conference on Advances in Wound Management*, (Ed. by K.G. Harding, C. Dealey, G. Cherry, F. Gottrup), 153. Macmillan Magazines Ltd, London.

McLaren, S.M.G. (1992) Nutrition and wound healing. In *Proceedings of the 1st Conference on Advances in Wound Management*, (Ed. by K.G. Harding, D.L. Leaper, T.D. Turner), 67–78. Macmillan Magazines Ltd, London.

Milward, P. (1993) How to manage pressure sores in the community, *British Journal of Nursing*, **2**, 488–92.

National Pressure Ulcer Advisory Panel (1989) Pressure ulcers: incidence, economics, risk assessment. Concensus Development Conference Statement, *Decubitus*, **2**, 24–8.

Norton, D., Exton-Smith, A.N. and Mclaren, R. (1975) *An Investigation of Geriatric Nursing Problems in Hospital*. Churchil Livingstone, Edinburgh.

Nyquist, R. and Hawthorn, P.J. (1987) The prevalence of pressure sores within an area health authority, *Journal of Advanced Nursing*, **12**, 183–7.

Patel, U.H., Jones, J.T., Babbs, C.F., Bourland, J.D. and Graber, G.P. (1993) Evaluation of five specialised support surfaces by the use of a pressure sensitive mat, *Decubitus*, **6**, 28–31, 34, 36–7.

Preston, K. W. (1988) Positioning for comfort and pressure relief: the 30 degree alternative, *Care-Science and Practice*, **6**, 116–19.

Roe, B.H., Cullum, N.A. and Hamer, C.L. (1995) Patients' perceptions of chronic leg ulceration. In *Leg Ulcers: Nursing Management* (Ed. by N.A. Cullum and B.H. Roe), Scutari, Harrow.

Rogers, M.A. (1994) Healing – the patient's perspective. In *Proceedings of the 3rd Conference on Advances in Wound Management* (Ed. by K.G. Harding, C. Dealey, G. Cherry and Finn Gottrup), 155. Macmillan Magazines Ltd, London.

Stapleton, M. (1986) Preventing pressure sores. An evaluation of three products, *Geriatric Nursing*, **6**, 23–5.

Thomas, S. (1990) *Wound Management and Dressings*. Pharmaceutical Press, London.

Touche Ross and Co. (1993) *The Costs of Pressure Sores – Report to the Department of Health*. Touche Ross and Co., London.

Turner, T.D., Cockbill, S.M.E. and Thomas, S. (1994) A survey of the current and continuing educational status of wound management in community nursing. In *Proceedings of the 3rd Conference on Advances in Wound Management* (Ed. by K.G. Harding, C. Dealey, G. Cherry, F. Gottrup), 147–9. Macmillan Magazines Ltd, London.

Tuttiett, S. (1990) *Wheelchair Cushions. Summary Report*. HMSO, London.

Waterlow, J. (1985) A risk assessment card, *Nursing Times*, **81**, 49–55.

Williams, C. (1991) Comparing Norton and Medley, *Nursing Times*, **87**, 66–8.

Winter, G.D. (1962) Formation of the scab and the rate of epithelialisation of superficial wounds in the skin of the young domestic pig, *Nature*, **193**, 293–4.

Young, J. (1990) Pressure sores – do mattresses work? *The Lancet*, **336**, 182–3.

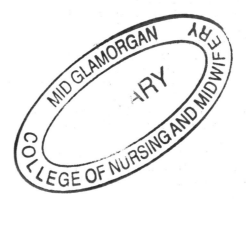

6

Management of Leg Ulcers

E. Andrea Nelson

6.1 INTRODUCTION

'Ulcers on the leg form a very extensive and important class of diseases ... The treatment of such cases is generally looked upon as an inferior branch of practice; an unpleasant and inglorious task where much labour must be bestowed, and little honour gained'.

This quotation from *The Inquirer* (1805) shows that the image of leg ulcers has not changed in nearly 200 years. The care of patients with leg ulcers is largely the responsibility of the community nurse; around 75% of leg ulcer patients are cared for totally within the community (Callam *et al.*, 1985). GPs often delegate assessment and treatment decisions to nurses (Ertl, 1991), and few patients are cared for at specialist leg ulcer clinics, whether in the community or the hospital.

A significant proportion of district nurse time is spent looking after patients with leg ulcers (Nicholls, 1990). Community nurses often work alone without the opportunity to share knowledge with their peers or discuss treatment options. Many patients receive little or no compression (Stockport Health Authority, 1990), the mainstay of the treatment of venous ulcers (Browse *et al.*, 1988). This may be due to lack of knowledge or the acknowledgement that inappropriate compression bandaging can be disastrous (Callam *et al.*, 1987). Accurate assessment is the key to successful treatment (Dale & Gibson, 1992). Once a nursing diagnosis is made, realistic aims and goals can be set, and appropriate referrals to medical agencies can be initiated. The nurse does not establish a medical diagnosis but can identify those ulcers which require referral.

Incidence and prevalence of leg ulcers

Two major UK studies of the pattern of leg ulceration in the community have indicated that the point prevalence of ulceration (active ulcers at the time of survey) is between 1.5 and 1.8 per thousand adults (Dale *et al.*, 1983; Cornwall *et al.*, 1986). These figures agree with estimates for other developed countries (Widmer, 1978; Andersson *et al.*, 1984). The proportion of the population likely to suffer from leg ulceration has been estimated to be 1% of adults, and over 3% of the elderly (Callam *et al.*, 1985). The majority of ulcers are due to venous disease (70–75%), the rest being due to peripheral vascular disease (10–15%), diabetes (5%), and rheumatoid disease (10%). Rarer causes of ulceration include sickle cell anaemia and neoplasm.

Although leg ulceration is often described as a disease of elderly women, 50% of patients have their first ulcer before the age of 65. The ratio of males to females is equal under the age of 40, although eventually the women outnumber the men by 3 to 1. A large number of patients suffer from recurrent ulceration. The rate of recurrence is high, up to 70% in 12 months (Monk & Sarkany, 1982).

The cost of leg ulcers

The single largest cost is the time of the community nurse. Although there are pressures to minimise the cost of products used, this may be a false economy if the healing of the ulcer is delayed or if additional visits are required. A survey of district nurse visits in one area showed that 70% of ulcers were dressed more than once a week (Lees & Lambert, 1992). The annual cost to the NHS has been estimated at £300 million (Laing, 1992). This does not include the loss of productivity due to illness. Nurses witness the personal costs of leg ulceration: pain, immobility, odour, altered self-perception, and isolation.

6.2 ANATOMY AND PHYSIOLOGY

The arterial system

The arterial system delivers blood from the heart to the capillaries via a network of arteries and arterioles. Arterial inflow can be disrupted by:

- poor pump function (left ventricular failure);
- arterial narrowing or obstruction (arteriosclerosis);
- inflammation of the smaller arterioles (arteritis).

Nursing interventions may reduce the metabolic demands but medical referral is essential to treat the underlying pathology. Signs of arterial insufficiency include shiny, hairless skin and slow capillary bed refilling (assessed after depressing the nail bed).

Symptoms of arterial insufficiency include intermittent claudication in which metabolic supply is only compromised during exercise, producing a sharp pain in the legs which is relieved on resting. Later on the pain occurs even at rest, and sitting with the feet dependent to increase arterial inflow relieves the situation temporarily, but eventually the tissues cannot be maintained and ulceration occurs. The nursing care of patients aims to educate them about the cause of ulceration, to reduce pain and likelihood of infection, and the impact on the patient's life. Arterial disease is normally progressive and healing the ulcer is likely only in the early stages of the disease.

The venous system

The heart propels blood distally, but a 'pump' is required to return blood upwards against the flow of gravity. This pump is made up of the calf muscle pump and the foot pump.

There are two systems of veins in the legs, the deep veins and the superficial veins. The long and short saphenous veins lie superficially, over the muscle fascia and collect blood from the capillary beds. They drain into the deep system, the popliteal and femoral veins, via perforating veins which literally perforate the calf muscle. The one-way valves in all these veins ensure that flow is from the superficial to the deep system and from the foot towards the heart.

When the calf muscle contracts it distorts the deep veins thus forcing blood upwards, retrograde flow being prevented by the valves. On relaxing, the lower pressure in the emptied vein encourages flow from the distal section of vein (Fig. 6.1).

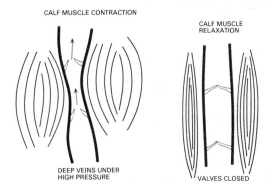

Figure 6.1 Normal calf muscle pump.

These mechanisms all rely on the patency of the venous valves. When the valves are incompetent due to damage, inherited weakness or vein wall distortion, reflux occurs, the veins become distended and the intravascular pressure increases (Fig. 6.2).

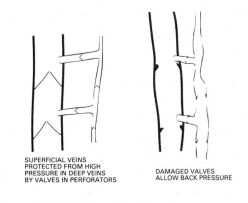

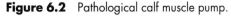

Figure 6.2 Pathological calf muscle pump.

Intravascular pressure also increases if the deep vein is obstructed, for example, by a thrombosis. The resulting venous hypertension, which is most marked during ambulation, causes venous ulceration.

6.3 PROCESS OF ULCERATION

Venous ulceration

Theories of ulceration try to account for experimental findings. The Fibrin Cuff Theory (Browse & Burnand, 1982) and the White Cell Trapping Theory (Coleridge-Smith *et al.*, 1988) are among the two most recent theories.

The Fibrin Cuff Theory

Increased venous hypertension leads to capillary hypertension and this causes increased capillary permeability. Leaked molecules such as fibrin are deposited around the capillary, and form a barrier to the diffusion of oxygen, nutrients and waste products. The fibrin is responsible for the stiffness of the tissues in the gaiter area of patients with chronic venous insufficiency. Red blood cell leakage into the interstitial space is followed by the deposition of the iron pigment haemosiderin in the gaiter area of the leg, thus accounting for the brown staining seen here. The term lipodermatosclerosis is used to describe the pigmented, indurated skin (Fig. 6.3).

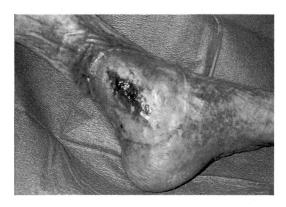

Figure 6.3   Lipodermatosclerosis.

The subcutaneous tissues are starved of oxygen, bathed in waste products and die. Graduated compression reduces the number of fibrin cuffs by enhancing fibrinolytic activity and reducing capillary filtration.

White Cell Trapping Theory

This hypothesis has been generated by the observation that white cells appear to become trapped in dependent legs. The deficit in white cells increases with the severity of venous disease. The white cells are 'washed out' when the leg is elevated but in patients with venous disease this takes much longer. White cells discharge their contents of proteolytic enzymes when they become trapped in capillaries, thus causing tissue necrosis. External graduated compression increases blood cell velocity and reduces the proportion of cells trapped.

External graduated compression heals venous ulcers by reducing ambulatory venous hypertension. Alternative ways of accomplishing this include prolonged bed rest and surgical correction of the venous abnormality.

Arterial ulcers

These ulcers are due to arterial insufficiency. This may be due to narrowing or obstruction of the arteries. The metabolic demand of the tissues is greater than the supply and thus the tissues ulcerate or die. Conservative measures cannot restore the impaired blood flow and nursing care consists of reducing the metabolic demands of the limb by keeping the ulcer warm and moist and protecting the skin from further damage from trauma or infection. Educating the patient may arrest deterioration of arterial supply, for example, by increasing exercise tolerance and reducing smoking. Pain control is an important part of the management of these patients (see Chapter 7).

Diabetic ulcers

Factors associated with ulceration in diabetics include arterial insufficiency, neuropathy, retinopathy, hammer toes, and decreased sensation (Holewski *et al.*, 1989). There may be concurrent venous disease but compression bandaging should not be applied because of the possibility of neuropathy and arterial insufficiency. Healing will be dependent, to a great extent, on the management of the diabetes. For further information see Chapter 10.

Rheumatoid ulcers

Patients with rheumatoid disease have an increased risk of leg ulceration although it is unclear whether this is due to the arthropathy and loss of function of the calf muscle pump, or to vasculitis. Cawley (1987) suggests that ulceration may be due to a combination of factors including: ankle joint dysfunction; vasculitis; venous insufficiency; arteriosclerosis; infection; neuropathy; trauma; pressure and deformity. If there is vasculitis or arteriosclerosis present, then compression bandaging is contraindicated. A nursing assessment will not reveal these and therefore support or compression bandaging is not recommended unless expressly requested by specialist medical staff.

In theory, both diabetic and rheumatoid patients may benefit from non-elastic compression as it exerts pressure on the limb only during standing or ambulation. At rest the sub-bandage pressure falls markedly and therefore patients with mildly impaired circulation are less likely to suffer skin damage. These non-elastic bandages, e.g. Rosidal K (Vernon-Carus, UK), are not available on prescription. The combination of a paste bandage and a support bandage (e.g. Elastocrepe, Smith and Nephew) might offer similar benefits; however, the decision to apply compression to limbs with concomitant diabetes or rheumatoid disease depends on a medical assessment.

Stages of healing

It is important to recognise these stages as ulcer progress can be assessed both in terms of the stage of healing reached and the size of the ulcer. Dressing selection also depends on the tissue present in the ulcer bed.

Necrosis

Once the tissues start to break down, dead cells need to be removed before healing can occur. If blood supply is severely reduced then the dead tissue is not broken down by macrophages and remains in place while it dies. This necrotic tissue is dry and black. Arterial ulcers and infected ulcers may go through a necrotic phase.

Slough

When tissues are digested by scavenging cells, the combination of dead cells, exudate and phagocytic cells is seen as slough, usually yellow and soft in appearance, on the wound surface. All ulcers normally go through a sloughy phase. The presence of slough does not mean that infection is present.

Granulation

Once the underlying reason for the cell breakdown has been reversed the process of healing by secondary intention can take place. Pink granulation tissue forms on the base of the ulcer to make up any depth deficit and once this has been achieved epithelialisation can start. Over granulation occurs when the new tissues have filled the deficit and continue to replicate so that they are proud of the surface.

Epithelialisation

New epithelium grows over the granulation tissue usually starting at the ulcer edge, seen as pink, shiny skin. Islands of epithelium may also start from hair follicles, appearing as white or pale pink dots in the pink/red granulation tissue.

Wound maturation

Once the ulcer has healed the covering skin continues to mature for 6–12 months. During this time the random matrix of collagen fibres which gives the skin its strength are realigned to form a well ordered structure. The patient must be aware of how fragile the skin is and how to protect it from trauma, for example, by moisturising it.

6.4 GUIDANCE FOR PRACTICE – ASSESSMENT OF LEG ULCERS

Assessing the whole person

This assessment will help towards a diagnosis and also identify factors which may predispose the patient to ulceration or delay healing.

The general assessment should include a record of:

- Age
- Sex

- Social situation
- Occupation
- Family history
- Psychological status
- Mobility
- Diet
- Obesity
- Smoking habits.

The medical history should include a record of:

- Circulatory problems such as varicose veins or phlebitis
- Vascular surgery
- Deep vein thrombosis (indicative of venous disease)
- Hypertension
- Myocardial infarction
- Stroke
- Intermittent claudication
- Diabetes
- Rheumatoid disease
- Current medication.

Urinalysis should be performed to rule out undiagnosed diabetes or to assess control, and blood screening for rheumatoid factor will identify rheumatoid disease. Measurement of the blood pressure is useful to screen for arterial disease.

Assessing the leg

The state of the patient's circulation is reflected in the state of the patient's skin. Hard, pigmented skin, lipodermatosclerosis, is suggestive of venous disease, as is the presence of distended capillaries in the region of the medial malleolus, called ankle flare (see Fig. 6.3). Cool, hairless, shiny skin, and toenails which regain their colour only slowly after the release of pressure are suggestive of arterial disease (see Fig. 6.4).

Palpation of strong dorsalis and posterior tibial foot pulses suggests adequate arterial supply although the small vessel disease in diabetics and those suffering from rheumatoid disease will not necessarily be revealed by investigation of the pulses, whether by palpation or doppler ultrasound assessment. Patients with an absent or weak pulse should be referred for a further assessment before being treated with compression.

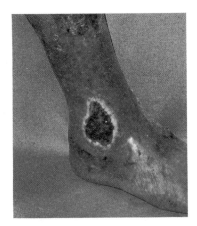

Figure 6.4 Arterial leg ulcer.

Assessing the ulcer

A detailed record of the ulcer's characteristics is essential for effective evaluation of progress and it may provide clues as to ulcer aetiology:

Site
Venous ulcers are generally found in the gaiter area of the leg. Arterial ulcers may also occur in this area but the presence of isolated ulcers on the foot is characteristic of arterial or diabetic ulceration.

Onset and duration
Venous ulcers tend to progress slowly whilst arterial involvement is usually indicated by very rapid development. An ulcer history which started when the patient was under 60 is suggestive of venous rather than arterial disease.

Size
The size of an ulcer can be recorded by tracing onto tracing grids, acetate film or polythene (use a clear plastic bag and discard side in contact with the ulcer). Measurement of length and width and subsequent calculation of ulcer area and photography are also useful. The ulcer should be assessed regularly, for example once a month, to monitor progress.

Appearance and depth
Venous ulcers are often large and shallow with a poorly defined edge. Small, deep and well defined ulcers are more likely to have an arterial component.

Oedema
With venous ulceration the generalised oedema often becomes worse during the day. Oedema associated

with arterial ulceration is more likely to be localised. Oedema affecting the toes is indicative of lymphatic disease.

Pain

The pain of venous ulcers may be associated with infection or oedema and can be helped by systemic treatment of any infection, elevation, and good graduated compression. Pain in these ulcers may be most common when the ulcer is new as tissue breakdown is still occurring. Arterial ulcers tend to be more painful and this is exacerbated by elevation and exercise. Patients may report that they need to hang their legs out of bed at night to relieve the pain. The patient with a venous ulcer may report having to get out of bed at night with a cramp pain which responds to walking or standing on a cold surface rather than ischaemic pain which is exacerbated by walking.

Ulcer base

The appearance of the ulcer base – necrosis, slough, granulation or epithelium – documents the ulcer progress. It is quite normal for more than one type of tissue to be present at any one time, in which case an outline of the ulcer areas is useful.

6.5 GUIDANCE FOR PRACTICE – TREATMENT OF LEG ULCERS

Cleansing

The purpose of cleaning an ulcer is to remove excess pus, slough, exudate and dressing residue. The ulcer surface is invariably colonised with bacteria and cleansing will have no influence on this. Rubbing the ulcer surface will damage granulation tissue and disturb the healing process. Warm saline irrigation of the ulcer is sufficient. Some centres use lined buckets filled with plain, warm tap water and combine the ulcer cleansing with cleaning the surrounding skin. There has not been a systematic study of the use of tap water although there are no reports of infection. This is an easy way to remove remnants of previous creams, dressings, and dry skin scales and is appreciated by patients.

Dressings

There is no evidence from clinical trials that the choice of primary dressing influences the healing rate of leg ulcers. This may be due to the poor quality of the trials and the fact that the correction of the underlying aetiology is the most important determinant of ulcer healing (just as in the treatment of pressure sores the most important step is the relief of pressure). The choice of a modern wound dressing will influence patient comfort, skin condition and the ulcer stage. According to Morgan (1987) the dressing selected should be:

- capable of maintaining a warm, moist, micro-environment conducive to healing;
- capable of absorbing the exudate away from the surrounding skin;
- non-adherent;
- non-toxic;
- non-allergenic;
- non-sensitising.

Paste bandages are used as a skin dressing and to augment compression but their constituents can cause allergic reaction and the initial application needs to be followed up with a visit or call from the nurse in 24 hours to check for any allergic reaction (Cameron, 1990).

Dressings should be changed as little as possible, preferably weekly, in order not to disturb granulation tissue. The dressing may need to be changed more frequently when there is infection, strike through, excessive slough, for patient comfort, or when particular dressings are used, e.g. hydrogels (Intrasite, Smith and Nephew).

Topical applications of creams, sprays or antibiotic powders should not be used as they have no proven value in ulcer healing and are a major cause of allergic skin reactions (Morgan, 1987). Silver sulphadiazine (Flamazine, Smith and Nephew) is useful against pseudomonas infection in conjunction with systemic antibiotics. Topical metronidazole has been shown to reduce the odour of ulcers but there is no evidence that it influences healing. Povidone-iodine has a wide spectrum of activity against most major pathogens (bacteria, fungi), e.g. Inadine (Johnson and Johnson).

Compression

Graduated, sustained compression is essential for the

ambulatory treatment of venous ulcers. Intermittent compression has been shown to accelerate the healing of venous ulcers but the patient cannot carry on with normal activities and so this is likely to be reserved for intractable ulcers or inpatient treatment.

Pain

Patients with leg ulcers report that pain is a significant problem (Hamer *et al.*, 1994). A pain scale should be used to monitor pain – any increase may indicate infection, increasing oedema or ischaemia. The cause of the pain should be treated with antibiotics, compression or rest and analgesia. A short period of bed rest may be required if the pain continues. Pain around the gaiter area may cause the patient to keep the ankle fixed in position but the mobility of this joint is necessary for the function of the calf muscle pump and therefore patients should be encouraged to mobilise the ankle. Arterial ulcers require an occlusive dressing and thermal insulation as ulcer desiccation or cooling increases the metabolic demand thus causing pain.

Infection

There is no need to take routine bacteriological swabs as these will reveal that the ulcer surface is colonised with skin flora. Clinical infection is present when there is increased pain, exudate, purulent slough, and cellulitis (see Fig. 6.5). In this situation a bacteriology swab should be taken to determine antibiotic therapy. The dressing may require more frequent changes due to the increased exudate.

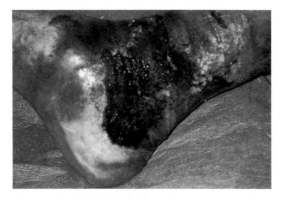

Figure 6.5 Infected leg ulcer.

Skin problems

Eczema is normally associated with venous ulceration and it may cause pain and irritation. The eczema and itch needs to be treated otherwise scratching of the leg will lead to further ulceration. Compression will reduce the eczema but there may be a need for short term therapy with dilute steroid preparations, e.g. hydrocortisone 1% ointment or cream. Dermatology referral may be required in some patients to treat the eczema and for patch testing.

Dry and hyperkeratotic skin can build up under bandages over time. These can be treated by washing the skin with plain water, and moisturising the skin with oil (e.g. arachis oil or olive oil) or 50:50 ointment (50% soft paraffin + 50% liquidparaffin). Other creams should be avoided as they often contain allergenic substances, e.g. lanolin or preservatives. Atrophie blanche (patches of white skin) are very poorly perfused and require protection from trauma. They are extremely likely to break down and should be carefully observed.

Posture and exercise

Patients with all kinds of ulcers should be encouraged to maintain joint mobility. Ankle mobility is particularly important for calf muscle function. Ask the patient to perform exercises for the ankle and toes, flexion and rotation, 50 times a day. Once ankle function is regained, check that the patient flexes the ankle during walking. The use of slippers encourages a poor, shuffling gait in which the leg flexes only at the hip, and should be discouraged. A pair of sensible shoes should be worn while the patient takes some exercise each day.

Leg elevation will aid the healing of venous ulcers. Ideally the heels should be higher than the hips. This can be achieved by using a high stool or leg rest, by lying on a sofa with the heels resting on the arm rests, or by going to bed for a rest in the afternoon. The degree of elevation possible depends on the patient's concurrent health. The end of the bed can be elevated by six inches to encourage venous return at night, although the health of a partner must also be taken into consideration. A firm pillow, bolster, brick, or old telephone directories placed between the mattress and the bed frame will elevate the lower portion of the bed. The patient should be advised not to stand still or sit still for long periods as this may cause oedema formation.

Prevention of recurrence

Recurrence is extremely likely unless the underlying pathology is treated, e.g. by surgery. For those who may not be suitable for surgery conservative measures must be used. Preventive measures should begin when the patient is first seen. This will increase the likelihood that healing will be achieved. Lifestyle changes will take time and the nurse is unlikely to have the time to see the patient frequently once the ulcer has healed. Ideally the patient should be seen regularly after healing to reinforce preventive measures and to treat any recurrence early.

Venous ulcers

Once venous ulcers are healed continued compression is essential. Compression hosiery is available on prescription in three classes according to the support provided. For the majority of patients class 2 or 3 below knee stockings are suitable. Patients with osteoarthritis of the knee or large varices around the knee may prefer stockings which include the knee. Higher compression (class 3) is more effective but compliance is better with moderate (class 2) compression. The highest class which the patient can apply, tolerate, and remove should be used. Measurements of the ankle and calf circumference and leg length are necessary to ensure the correct size is supplied. The stockings last between 4 and 6 months, if washed according to the manufacturers' instructions, before requiring refitting and re-supply. A small proportion of patients may not be able to remove or put on stockings and so they may need to remain in compression bandages which are changed weekly, or wear light support hosiery overnight (although this is not recommended by the stocking manufacturers). A frame which helps stocking application, the Medi Valet (Medi, UK), may help a number of patients or their carers. Some patients will be suitable for vein stripping surgery which may reduce the likelihood of recurrence and so referral to a surgeon should be considered.

Arterial ulcers

Reduction in smoking, improvement in diet, increasing mobility, and monitoring concurrent disease will aid healing as well as reducing recurrence. In the long term arterial reconstruction or sympathectomy may be necessary. Referral to a vascular surgeon is essential in the early stages of ulceration.

Summary

Prevention of ulcer recurrence should include:

- Protection of skin
- Compression hosiery for ulcers of venous origin
- Exercise and mobility
- Health education
- Surgical referral
- Continued observation.

6.6 GUIDANCE FOR PRACTICE – DOPPLER ULTRASOUND ASSESSMENTS

Assessing arterial circulation

The purpose of doppler ultrasound assessment is to determine whether compression can be applied to a leg. The calculation of an index, the ankle brachial pressure index (ABPI) or the resting pressure index (RPI), indicates whether arterial supply to the leg is significantly impaired. Doppler assessment is performed after the initial assessment, when it is thought that the ulcer is venous but confirmation is needed that arterial circulation to the limb is not impaired. It does not establish a diagnosis.

How to perform doppler assessment

Preparation of equipment
You will need a doppler ultrasound machine with an 8 MHz probe, water soluble gel, tissues, blood pressure cuff, recording documents, and calculator or chart to work out the ABPI (see Fig. 6.6).

Patient preparation
Explain to the patient the nature and purpose of the investigation. Provide sensory information to relieve stress (the arterial signal sounds like a dog barking). Preferably ask patient to lie supine for 5–10 minutes to allow blood pressure to stabilise. If this is not practical, e.g. if patient does not have a bed or cannot

Dopplex® Ankle Pressure Index Guide

Leg ulcers are commonly treated using compression therapy - bandages, stockings or Flowtron' Intermittent Compression. It is essential to establish signs of sufficient arterial supply prior to using compression therapy so enabling the most appropriate treatment. The Dopplex' Ankle Pressure Index (API) guide will assist you to quickly and efficiently identify any underlying circulatory problems.

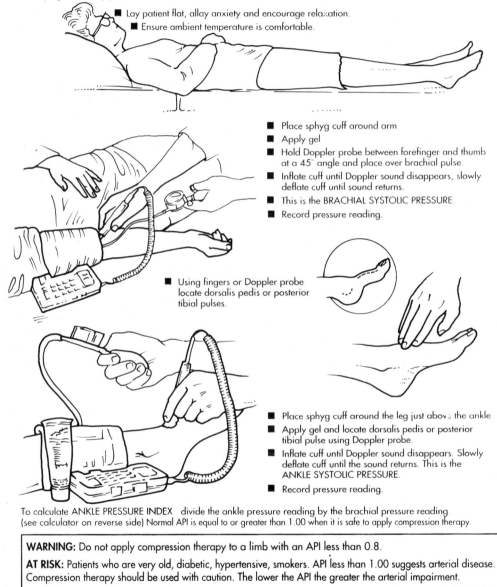

- Lay patient flat, allay anxiety and encourage relaxation.
- Ensure ambient temperature is comfortable.

- Place sphyg cuff around arm
- Apply gel
- Hold Doppler probe between forefinger and thumb at a 45° angle and place over brachial pulse.
- Inflate cuff until Doppler sound disappears, slowly deflate cuff until sound returns.
- This is the BRACHIAL SYSTOLIC PRESSURE.
- Record pressure reading.

- Using fingers or Doppler probe locate dorsalis pedis or posterior tibial pulses.

- Place sphyg cuff around the leg just above the ankle.
- Apply gel and locate dorsalis pedis or posterior tibial pulse using Doppler probe.
- Inflate cuff until Doppler sound disappears. Slowly deflate cuff until the sound returns. This is the ANKLE SYSTOLIC PRESSURE.
- Record pressure reading.

To calculate ANKLE PRESSURE INDEX divide the ankle pressure reading by the brachial pressure reading. (see calculator on reverse side) Normal API is equal to or greater than 1.00 when it is safe to apply compression therapy.

WARNING: Do not apply compression therapy to a limb with an API less than 0.8.

AT RISK: Patients who are very old, diabetic, hypertensive, smokers. API less than 1.00 suggests arterial disease. Compression therapy should be used with caution. The lower the API the greater the arterial impairment.

---

1. Moffatt C. The Charing Cross approach to venous ulcers *Nursing Standard* 1990; Dec 12, **5 No. 12**, 6-9. © Huntleigh Technology plc 1994
Huntleigh Nesbit Evans Healthcare

Figure 6.6   Ankle Pressure Index Guide. Source: *Dopplex Ankle Pressure Index Guide*, courtesy of Huntleigh Nesbit Evans Healthcare.

lie flat, ask patient to lie on a sofa, or sit in a chair with legs supported by a high foot stool.

Brachial systolic pressure measurement

Measure the brachial systolic pressure first so that the patient gets accustomed to the sound from the doppler ultrasound (or wear the headphones generally supplied). Measure systolic brachial pressure *of the arm on the same side as the ulcerated leg* using the ultrasound probe. In outline, the procedure is:

- Place cuff on upper arm.
- Insonate pulse.
- Inflate cuff until pulse is obliterated.
- Release cuff until first sound is heard and note cuff pressure at which this occurs.

Place cuff on upper arm

Place the cuff around the arm as for a normal blood pressure measurement, but keep the tubing away from the gel by putting the cuff on upside down.

Insonate pulse

Find the brachial pulse by palpation and apply ultrasound gel or water based lubricating gel, e.g. KY jelly, to the pulse site. Turn the doppler machine on. Place the 8 MHz probe lightly onto the gel at an angle of 45° to the skin and move the probe slowly in a circular pattern until you hear the definite 'thump, thump' of the arterial pulse (cf venous signal, a slow whoosh). Once you have located the pulse, keep the probe in the same spot but tilt it slowly to find the point at which the signal is at its loudest. Try to position your hand so that you can stabilise it on the patient's arm. Then, if the arm moves during the assessment, you will be able to keep the probe stable.

Inflate cuff until pulse is obliterated

Inflate the cuff while listening to the arterial signal. Keep the sphygmomanometer dial or mercury column near the probe so that you can see both at the same time. Watch the probe to confirm that you have not let it slip off position. Inflate until no signal is heard and then inflate another 10–20 mmHg.

Release cuff until pulse is heard and note cuff pressure at which this occurs

Let the cuff down slowly and note the reading at which the first 'thump' is heard. Then let the cuff down quickly – there is no diastolic reading. If the patient's pulse is slow or irregular you will have to let the cuff down very slowly to get an accurate reading. Practise with the probe in both left and right hands, as depending on your dexterity, strength and the type of sphygmomanometer available, you may prefer to inflate and deflate the cuff with the dominant hand and hold the probe in the non-dominant hand.

The leg blood pressure

This can be measured in the peroneal, dorsalis pedis (DP), posterior tibial (PT) and digital (toe) arteries. It is sufficient to measure the DP and PT pressures.

Place the cuff around the gaiter area of the leg. If the ulcer is in this area, cover it with a surgical pad, gauze swabs, plastic bag, waterproof dressing, or clean cling film to ensure that the cuff is not contaminated. Position the cuff upside down on the leg to keep the tubing away from the gel. If the patient is anxious about the cuff being inflated on the ulcer, either perform measurement first on the non-ulcerated leg to demonstrate what it may feel like, or place the cuff higher up the leg over the calf muscle. In the latter case a larger cuff might be needed. The procedure may be less comfortable when done on the calf as the muscle is compressed. If the ulcer is arterial the whole procedure may be uncomfortable or painful. Be prepared to abandon the investigation when patients complain of extreme pain on inflating the cuff as they are unlikely to comply with compression.

The DP artery runs down the front of the foot. It is palpable in the mid line of the foot above the foot arch and it can also be insonated here. It runs down to between the first and second toes and it can be insonated here too, although it cannot be palpated here. The advantage of placing the probe in this groove is that it is less likely to slip off the pulse accidentally. The probe tends to slip off the pulse easily on the top of the foot. You should practise insonating the pulse at both positions as in some patients only one may be heard. It helps to stabilise your hand on the patient's foot.

The PT artery runs down the back of the leg, behind the medial malleolus. It can be palpated and insonated at a point approximately half way between the point of the heel and the medial malleolus. Ask the patient to dorsiflex the foot as this makes the pulse easier to feel. Measure the PT pressure in the same way as the DP and brachial pulses. Record DP and PT pressure.

Ankle brachial pressure index or resting pressure index

To calculate the ABPI/RPI take the higher leg pressure (DP or PT) and divide it by the arm pressure using a calculator. To remember this calculation (leg over arm) note that ABPI starts with AB, and the ratio is A (for ankle) over B (for brachial). A normal RPI is around 1, that means the blood pressure of the arm and the leg are approximately the same. A low RPI, say around 0.6, indicates that the arterial supply to the leg is significantly impaired. An index below 0.8 (or 0.9, depending on centre) indicates that it is no longer safe to apply compression.

Points to remember about the ABPI

- It cannot tell you the condition of the arterioles which may be inflamed (because of inflammatory diseases such as rheumatoid arthritis).
- It may be misleading if the leg pressure is high, e.g. > 200, as this indicates atherosclerosis. Again the condition of the smaller arterioles is unknown but there may be arterial disease present.
- It decreases with age, therefore a new assessment must be made if the ulcer is not healing or it is a year since last measurement.
- A patient may have an 'arterial' and a contra lateral 'venous' leg, therefore accurate assessment and documentation is vital.
- The ABPI merely forms part of an assessment. If it indicates that a compression bandage can be applied then the nurse's assessment skills are required every time the bandage is removed. Do not place more weight on the ABPI alone than your own assessment of ulcer progress or skin condition.

Ultrasound assessment of veins

The doppler ultrasound can also be used to assess the patency and competency of the veins. The doppler probe is used to insonate the veins while the muscle distal to it is pressed to cause the blood to flow proximally in the vein. If the vein is patent, then a signal is heard while pressing the vein. If the valves are competent, when the muscle is released there is no distal flow and thus no signal is heard. A biphasic signal indicates reflux (incompetence). Community nurses are unlikely to be asked to perform this investigation.

6.7 GUIDANCE FOR PRACTICE – COMPRESSION THERAPY

Compression can be provided by hosiery, shaped tubular or roller bandages. Each has advantages and disadvantages (see Table 6.1) but the basic principles by which they exert their pressure are the same. Once the principles are understood you can tailor the compression to the individual patient.

Compression hosiery

Compression stockings are used to prevent ulcer recurrence but they can also be used to provide the graduated compression necessary for the healing of venous leg ulcers. They are classified as class 1, 2 or 3 depending on the amount of pressure they exert at the ankle. The compression of class 2 or 3 will be necessary to heal ulcers. It is recommended that the stockings are removed at night and therefore patients must be able to apply and remove them or have someone else to do this for them. If patients are able to don and doff them it may also be possible to teach them to change their own dressings.

Elasticated tubular bandages

These bandages are only useful in the treatment of leg ulcers if they are graduated, e.g. Flexishape (Smith and Nephew) or Shaped Support Bandage, SSB (Seton). If used on their own to provide support, a double layer is required. They can be used over compression bandages to augment the pressure applied and to help keep the bandages in place. Patients who complain that their bandages become tight in the evening due to oedema, may be instructed on how to remove and re-apply them first thing in the morning. This prevents patients from removing the whole bandage. Bandages are available in a range of sizes, in full and half leg versions and can be hand washed. They should not be pulled on, but rolled up into a doughnut shape and then rolled onto the leg. The fabric can be over-extended at the front of the foot as the tubular fabric cannot accommodate the large radius of the heel. If there is any sign of pressure damage at this point the tension may be relieved by cutting a small hole in the fabric.

Straight bandages, e.g. Tubigrip (Seton), are not

Table 6.1 Comparison of compression devices.

Compression bandages	
Advantages	*Disadvantages*
Compression can be varied.	Skill required to apply effectively.
If washable, they have a low unit cost.	If not washable can be costly.
Can be used on all shapes of leg and ulcer.	
Available on prescription.	

Compression stockings	
Advantages	*Disadvantages*
Known level of compression applied.	Needs measurement and fitting.
No skill required to apply.	Needs to be removed at night.
Aids self-care and independence.	Unsuitable for extensive/exuding lesions.
Lasts 4–6 months (cost effective).	Requires remeasuring and fitting as oedema resolves.
Available on prescription.	Not suitable for arthritic patients.

Shaped support bandage (Flexishape/Tubigrip SSB)	
Advantages	*Disadvantages*
Easy to apply.	Not available on prescription.
Layers 'build up' compression.	Lasts only a few washes.
Can be used over bandages for retention.	Can be tight at front of foot.

suitable as they produce a tourniquet at the calf if they fit at the ankle, or are loose at the ankle if they fit at the calf.

Compression bandages

Thomas (1990) has classified bandages according to their performance in mechanical tests. These give information on the strength of the bandage on application and its ability to maintain pressure as shown in Table 6.2.

It is essential to use a bandage for the purpose for which it was designed:

- *Retention bandages* are designed to keep dressings in place. They exert very little pressure on a limb and are conformable.
- *Support bandages* are designed to stop oedema from forming or to support joints. They can be stretched only a small distance before they 'lock out' at which point they cannot be stretched any further. The majority of crepe bandages are support, not compression, bandages.
- *Compression bandages* can apply *and retain* pressure on a limb and are classified as light, moderate, high and extra high compression bandages depending on the amount of pressure they exert.

Table 6.2 Thomas' classification of bandages.

Bandage type	Proprietary example
(1) Conforming stretch	Easifix, J-Fast, Slinky, Tensofix
(2) Light support	Crepe BP, Elastocrepe, Elastoplast
(3a) Light compression (14–17 mmHg at ankle)	J-Plus, K-Crepe
(3b) Moderate compression (18–24 mmHg at ankle)	Veinopress
(3c) High compression (25–35 mmHg at ankle)	Setopress, Tensopress
(3d) Extra high compression (36–60 mmHg at ankle)	Blue Line

Bandage application

Factors which control the amount of pressure on a limb are the choice of bandage, the tension generated, the number of layers of bandage and the shape of the limb. Two layers of bandage will exert twice the pressure of one layer, therefore to achieve an even, graduated pressure along a limb there needs to be a consistent layer of bandage all the way along the limb. A bandage applied to a limb with a small radius will exert a higher pressure than when applied to a large radius. This is because the tension force is not spread over a wide area and is concentrated. An analogy is the discomfort felt when carrying a heavy bag on one finger rather than the whole hand.

These factors are summarised by Laplace's law:

- Pressure (P) is proportional to tension (T).
- Pressure is proportional to the number of layers used (N).
- Pressure is inversely proportional to radius of curvature (R).

$$P = k \, T \, N / R \text{ (k is a constant)}$$

Thus the pressure applied to the leg can be varied by choice of bandage, modifying the tension used, padding the leg (to increase the radius), and using a different number of layers. Correct bandage placement with a 50% overlap will ensure that there is even coverage of the leg, with two layers of bandage all the way up the leg. Other overlaps may be used only if the result is an even coverage of the leg, i.e.

- 3 layers require a 66% overlap or 6.66 cm on a 10 cm bandage
- 4 layers require a 75% overlap or 7.5 cm on a 10 cm bandage
- 5 layers require an 80% overlap or 8 cm on a 10 cm bandage.

There are bandages with lines to guide 50% and 66% overlaps but other overlaps are seldom used as they are difficult to estimate and there are other easier ways to increase the pressure, e.g. using an additional bandage, selecting a stronger bandage, using a greater extension.

Bandage extension is specified in some bandages either by use of symbols, e.g. rectangles which become square at the correct extension, or by recommending the percentage extension for a range of leg sizes. The first type of bandages, e.g. Setopress (Seton, UK), are supplied with detailed instructions. For the latter type the bandage extension is measured as follows:

- Mark a bandage along its centre line at 10 cm intervals using a marker pen.
- Apply the bandage with marks outermost in a spiral with 50% overlap.
- After application measure the distance between successive marks at the ankle, gaiter and calf.
- Calculate the bandage extension thus:

$$\text{extension (\%)} = 10 \times (\text{new distance} - 10)$$
e.g. if new separation of marks = 12 cm,
$$\text{extension} = 10 \times (12 - 10) = 10 \times 2 = 20\%$$
or if new separation of marks = 14.5 cm, extension $= 10 \times (14.5 - 10) = 10 \times (4.5) = 45\%$

The extension should not increase up the leg, it should remain the same or decrease up the leg. For example,

extension around ankle = 45%,
extension, around gaiter = 30%,
extension around calf = 30%.

The commonest mistake is the production of a tourniquet at the gaiter or calf by overextending the bandage or by applying more layers here.

Bandaging techniques

In all these bandaging techniques the leg is covered from the base of the metatarsals to the tibial plateau. Leaving out areas leads to oedema formation. The grossly oedematous leg is particularly vulnerable to bandage damage and it is recommended that oedema is reduced by a period of bed rest prior to application of a compression bandage. In order to allow the patient the maximum range of motion of the ankle joint, the leg should be bandaged with the ankle in a neutral position. Bandaging for a venous ulcer is usually done with the patient seated and the leg dependent.

Simple spiral

This is the simplest technique and the majority of elastic bandages are applied in this way. Other methods, e.g. figure of eight, are based on this and so it will be described in detail; for the advantages of these two methods see Table 6.3.

Table 6.3 Comparison of bandaging techniques.

Advantages of spiral bandages	Advantages of figure of eight bandages
Simple to apply.	Provides more compression than the spiral method.
Recommended for strong compression bandages.	Bandages are less likely to slip down the leg.
Patients may be trained to reapply their own bandages.	Easier to apply on an unusual shaped leg.

It is usual to have a 50% overlap, so the leg is covered with two layers of bandage from ankle to knee.

The foot
This part of the bandaging remains the same whether a spiral or figure of eight technique is being used. The layers of bandage on the foot are kept to a minimum so that patients will be able to wear their usual footwear and be able to walk normally in order to utilise the calf pump. Do not use the extension recommended for the rest of the leg because the bony foot will not tolerate high pressures over the thin skin, and because support is also provided by footwear.

- The first turn encircles the ball of the foot and anchors the bandage in place.
- The next turn takes the bandage to the point of the heel and back to the front of the foot ready to cover the arch of the foot with the next turn.
- The last turn encircles the rest of the foot and returns to the Achilles tendon from where the straight part of the leg can be approached (Fig. 6.7).

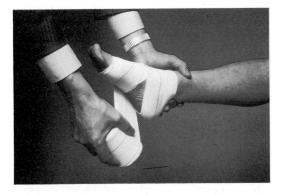

Figure 6.7 Bandaging the ankle.

The rest of the leg
At this point extend the bandage to its required extension.

- Unroll sufficient bandage to wrap around the leg.
- Extend it to the required extension.
- Place it on the leg so that 50% of the previous turn is covered (Fig. 6.8).

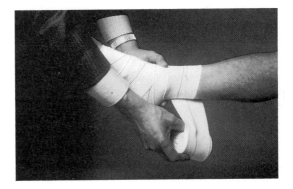
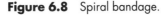

Figure 6.8 Spiral bandage.

When using cohesive or adhesive bandages, release the bandage from the roll and then relax the bandage fully before extending it to the required extension, otherwise it is easy to apply these bandages at full stretch straight from the roll. Transfer the bandage from one hand to the other keeping the bandage away from the leg. This will achieve an even extension and overlap up the leg to the tibial plateau, where the bandage is finished off so that the knee joint is not impeded. In obese patients the knee joint may be difficult to locate so ask the patient to bend the knee in order to determine its position. Any excess bandage is cut off rather than wound around the leg because it produces a tourniquet effect at the calf. Use adhesive tape to secure the bandage effectively. Pins or metal fasteners should not be used because they may damage the skin of either the bandaged or the other leg.

Figure of eight

The foot is covered in the same way as in the spiral technique above. The first turn of the bandage on the leg is applied up the lateral aspect of the leg, straight along the back of the leg and then downwards along the medial aspect. The next turn along the back of the leg is offset by $\frac{1}{2}$ bandage width and the following turns are placed accordingly. The pattern repeats up the leg to the tibial plateau (Fig. 6.9).

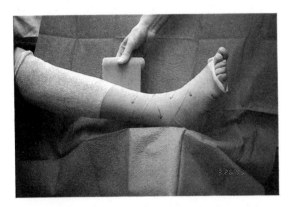

Figure 6.9   Figure of eight bandage.

Paste bandaging

These bandages can be used in conjunction with a compression bandage. They are a dressing and a skin treatment. They improve the maintenance of compression of some bandages and can augment the pressures achieved. The disadvantage of paste bandages is the high rate of allergy they cause, around 16% (Cameron, 1990). The application of a paste bandage for the first time should always be followed up by a visit or phone call from the nurse to check that there is no allergic reaction. These bandages are inelastic and are applied in such a manner that the leg does not become constricted by them due to swelling. One can apply them with frequent folds in the fabric or by cutting them into strips. Dale and Gibson (1992) recommend the former as the folds can be placed along the tibial crest as a protection from pressure damage. As this method requires consider-

able dexterity, the infrequent user may prefer to cut the bandage after every circumference of the leg.

Minimising pressure necrosis

Pressure damage can occur where there is localised high pressure or where a bandage has been applied to a leg with impaired arterial inflow or sensation. To minimise the chance of necrosis, therefore, the first safeguard is a thorough assessment. However, pressure damage can occur on any leg and therefore the skin should always be thoroughly inspected upon removing a bandage. The shape of the leg will determine which areas are liable to localised high pressure. From Laplace's law it is seen that pressure is greater at small radii of curvature, e.g. the tendon crests, malleoli, and shin bone. The foot may also be prone to damage as there is very little subcutaneous padding. Reducing the localised pressure on the foot can be achieved by reducing the bandage tension or using extra padding, although this may mean that footwear no longer fits. Very thin legs, with a circumference less than 18 cm, should be padded, have bandages applied at a lesser extension, or a weaker bandage selected.

Vulnerable areas can be protected by flattening the curvature of the leg using foam, gauze or orthopaedic padding materials. Red marks on these areas which do not disappear within a minute or two, or skin breaks, should be regarded as pressure damage. The principle of treating these is the same as for any pressure sore – reduce the pressure. If padding has not been successful then the diagnosis should be reviewed and the bandage tension reduced further or a less strong bandage chosen.

6.8 SUMMARY

The treatment of leg ulcers is a high cost high volume activity. A significant proportion of community nurses' time is spent looking after patients with leg ulcers.

It is important to assess and accurately diagnose the type of ulcer before treatment. External graduated compression is the treatment of choice in the management of venous ulcers. Arterial ulcers on the other hand require the nurse to reduce the metabolic demands of the limb by keeping the ulcer warm and moist and protecting the skin from further damage from trauma or infection. Educating the patient may arrest deterioration of the arterial supply, for example, by increasing exercise tolerance or reducing smoking. In patients with diabetic or rheumatoid ulcers compression bandaging is not recommended.

An important but often neglected element of community nursing intervention is the prevention of ulcer recurrence.

6.9 REFERENCES AND FURTHER READING

Andersson, E., Hansson, C., Swanbeck, G. (1984) Leg and foot ulcers. An epidemiological survey, *Acta Dermato-Venereologica* (Stockholm), **64**, 3, 227–32.

Browse, N.L. & Burnand, K.G. (1982) The cause of venous ulceration, *The Lancet*, **2**, 8292, 243–5.

Browse, N.L., Burnand, K.G. & Lea Thomas, M. (1988) *Diseases of the Veins: Pathology, Diagnosis and Treatment*. Edward Arnold, London.

Callam, M.J., Ruckley, C.V., Harper D.R. & Dale, J.J. (1985) Chronic ulceration of the leg: extent of the problem and provision of care, *British Medical Journal*, **290**, 6485, 1855–6.

Callam, M.J., Harper, D.R., Dale, J.J., Ruckley, C.V. (1987) Arterial disease in chronic leg ulceration: an underestimated hazard? Lothian and Forth Valley leg ulcer study. *British Medical Journal*, **294**, 6577, 929–31.

Cameron, J. (1990) Patch testing for leg ulcer patients, *Nursing Times*, (Wound Care Supplement), **86**, 25, 63–75.

Cawley, M.I. (1987) Vasculitis and ulceration in rheumatic diseases of the foot, *Baillieres Clinical Rheumatology*, **1**, 2, 315–33.

Coleridge-Smith, P.D., Thomas, P., Scurr, J.H. & Dormandy, J.A. (1988) Causes of venous ulceration: a new hypothesis, *British Medical Journal*, **296**, 1726–7.

Cornwall, J.V., Dore, C.J., Lewis, J.D. (1986) Leg ulcers: epidemiology and aetiology, *British Journal of Surgery*, **73**, 9, 693–6.

Dale J.J. & Gibson, B.(1992) Leg ulcer management, *Professional Nurse*, **7**, 11, 755–60.

Dale, J.J., Callam, M.J., Ruckley, C.V., Harper, D.R., Berrey, P.N. (1983) Chronic ulcers of the leg: a study of prevalence in a Scottish community, *Health Bulletin* (Edinburgh), **41**, 6, 310–4.

Ertl, P. (1991) *A Survey of Leg Ulcers Treated by District Nurses in the Eastbourne Health Authority*. Royal Society of Medicine Venous Forum, October 25.

Hamer, C., Cullum, N.A. & Roe, B.H. (1994) Patients' perceptions of chronic leg ulcers, *Journal of Wound Care*, **3**, 2, 99–101.

Holewski, J.J., Moss, K.M., Stess, R.M., Graf, P.M. & Grunfeld, C. (1989) Prevalence of foot pathology and lower extremity complications in a diabetic outpatient clinic. *Journal of the Rehabilitation Research and Development Service*, **26**, 3, 35–44.

Laing, W. (1992) *Chronic Venous Diseases of the Leg*. Office of Health Economics, London.

Lees, T.A. & Lambert, D.(1992) Prevalence of lower limb ulceration in an urban health district, *British Journal of Surgery*, **79**, 1032–1034.

Monk, B.E. & Sarkany, I. (1982) Outcome of treatment of venous stasis ulcers, *Clinical and Experimental Dermatology*, **7**, 4, 397–400.

Morgan, D. (1987) Leg ulcers. Guides to information, *Nursing Times*, **83**, 12, 53–4.

Nicholls, R. (1990) Leg ulcers: a study in the community, *Nursing Standard*, supplement, **3**, 7, 4–6.

Stockport Health Authority (1990) A description and discussion of the diagnosis and management of leg ulcers treated by staff working in Stockport Health Authority. Unpublished report.

The Inquirer (1805). What are the comparative advantages of the different modes for the treatment of ulcerated legs?, *Edinburgh Medical and Surgical Journal*, **1**, 187–93.

Thomas, S. (1990) Bandages and bandaging: the science behind the art, *Care Science & Practice*, **8**, 2, 56–60.

Widmer, L.K. (1978) *Peripheral Venous Disorders: Prevalence and Sociomedical Importance*. Hans Huber, Bern.

7

Management of Pain

Susie Wilkinson

7.1 INTRODUCTION

The management of pain poses a challenge to all health care professionals who are involved in the relief of pain and suffering caused by injury, illness or disease. The World Health Organisation 1986 recognises cancer pain relief as a health care priority because 70% of patients with cancer experience pain (Baines, 1984). As cancer is the second commonest cause of death and cancer patients spend 90% of their final year being cared for at home (Griffin, 1991) pain relief is a major concern for community nurses. Furthermore, with the advent of the NHS and Community Care Act 1990, earlier discharges from hospital, the use of minimal access surgery and patients' desire to be cared for at home, good pain management has become a priority for community nurses.

Despite major technical advances, inadequate treatment of pain is a persistent problem (Cohen, 1980; Donovan *et al.* 1987). Pain control is reported to be one of the most frustrating aspects of patient care and health care professionals inadequately assess and treat pain (Graflam, 1981; Donovan, 1985; Camp, 1988; Dalton, 1989). Community nurses recognise these difficulties and wish to develop more knowledge in this area so that they do not have to rely on clinical nurse specialists (Griffiths & Luker, 1994).

Patients' experiences of pain and nurses' attitudes towards pain and pain relief vary. Many nurses do not believe it is possible to achieve complete relief from pain. Most nurses do not use assessment tools and are unsure of how often to assess pain (Scott, 1992). Accurate pain assessment is essential for good pain control.

Pain is considered to be a very complex concept (Bourbonnais, 1981; Graflam, 1981). Atkinsanya (1985) maintains that as pain is,

' a totally subjective experience, it is questionable whether it is sensible to attempt a verbal definition which will be universally recognised.'

Despite this, definitions of pain have been attempted. Merskey (1986) describes it is

'an unpleasant sensory and emotional experience associated with actual or potential tissue damage or described in terms of such damage.'

Melzack & Wall (1988) argue that the term unpleasant is not enough but point out that this definition does recognise the link between injury and pain and also that pain has an emotional aspect. One definition which is now widely used does take into account the subjective and personal experience. This is McCaffrey's (1983) which states:

'Pain is whatever the experiencing person says it is and exists wherever he says it does.'

Pain is subjective, thus it can be concluded that each person learns the application of the word through experiences related to injury in early life. It is unquestionably a sensation in a part or parts of the body which is unpleasant and therefore has an emotional aspect.

Theories of pain

There are three main theories of pain transmission: specificity theory; pattern theory; and the gate theory. These are described below.

Specificity theory

Specificity theory was originally described by Descartes in 1644. The theory proposes that from specific pain receptors in the skin, impulses travel straight to the pain centre in the thalamus and cerebral cortex in the brain via the fast myelinated A delta fibres and slow unmyelinated C fibres through the lateral spinothalamic tract in the spinal cord. However, specific pain receptors have not been identified and furthermore the body does not always interpret certain stimuli as pain.

Pattern theory

Pattern theory suggests that pain is produced by intense stimulation at the skin producing patterns of nerve impulses. Pain results when the total output from the skin receptor cells exceeds a critical level (Latham, 1991). However, this theory does not explain the function of the spinal cord or the pain relief achieved by neurosurgical interventions.

The gate theory

The gate theory first described by Melzack and Wall in 1965 proposes that a mechanism in the substantia gelatinosa which caps the grey matter of the dorsal horn in the spinal cord is the essential site of control. The gate or a series of gates exists throughout the length of the spinal cord. Pain impulses can only pass through when the gate is open. Two types of nerves which transmit the impulses are relevant to the gate theory:

- A delta and C fibres which are narrow in diameter and conduct impulses from pain receptors at a slow rate.
- A beta fibres which are larger in diameter and conduct impulses like vibration pressure and warmth at a faster rate.

The gate is opened by impulses along the slow fibres but remains closed if the large diameter fast fibres are stimulated. This theory does offer some explanation of pain relief by acupuncture, massage and transcutaneous electrical nerve stimulation. These therapies all stimulate the fast fibres and therefore stop pain impulses being transmitted up the spinal cord. The gate theory is held to be the most credible pain theory to date.

Acute and chronic pain

Pain is either acute or chronic. Chronic pain is a dull continuous pain which can persist regularly for an indefinite period in comparison to acute pain (Hanks, 1983). Acute pain, usually from trauma or an operation, eventually eases off. The different characteristics of acute and chronic pain are shown in Table 7.1.

Cancer pain and terminal pain are considered to be chronic in nature. It is the management of chronic pain that community nurses are most frequently involved with.

Table 7.1 Features of acute and chronic pain.

Acute pain	Chronic pain
An event	A situation
Observable signs of discomfort are present.	Observable signs of discomfort decrease although pain intensity is unchanged.
It has a clear meaning.	It has no meaning.
The ending is predictable.	It is not possible to predict the end.
It usually involves responses from the autonomic nervous system (sweating, tachycardia, raised B/P, dilated pupils, increased respiratory rate).	Autonomic nervous system responses are absent.
The individual can be distracted.	It can occupy the individual's whole attention.
It often gets better.	It often gets worse.

The perception of pain

Two concepts that are useful in determining how pain is psychologically and physiologically perceived are pain threshold and pain tolerance:

- Pain threshold is the point at which the person first feels pain, that is the amount of a noxious stimulus that is necessary before an individual feels pain, for example, the amount of heat to the skin. Pain thresholds vary between individuals and within individuals.
- Pain tolerance refers to the amount of pain that a person can tolerate, which again varies between individuals and within individuals.

loss of sense of self worth, and of the meaning of life or a lack of love.

- Social pain which may be caused by the anticipated loss or loss of status, a change in role in the family, loss of independence or the inability to fulfil life's expectations.
- Physical pain which can be caused by the disease itself or problems related to the disease. Examples include the development of constipation or pressure sores, a sore mouth from chemotherapy, sore skin from radiotherapy, chronic post operative scar pain. There could also be a concurrent disorder, for example, osteoarthritis or angina.

Table 7.2 Factors affecting the pain threshold.

Threshold lowered	Threshold raised – relief of symptoms
Discomfort	Sleep
Insomnia	Rest
Fatigue	Sympathy
Anxiety	Understanding
Fear	Companionship
Anger	Diversional activity
Sadness	Reduction in anxiety
Depression	Elevation of mood
Boredom	Analgesics
Introversion	Anxiolitics
Mental isolation	Anti-depressants
Social abandonment	

Both these concepts can be affected by culture, religious beliefs and the cause of the pain. Twycross (1978) suggests that the factors shown in Table 7.2 greatly affect a person's pain threshold.

Total pain

Pain is no longer considered to be a single phenomenon, and Saunders (1964) described the concept of 'total pain' (Fig. 7.1). Total pain encompasses four aspects of pain:

- Emotional pain which may be caused by fear of impending death, anxiety, anticipatory grief, anger, depression, isolation and loneliness.
- Spiritual pain which may arise from loss of faith, a

7.2 GUIDANCE FOR PRACTICE – PAIN ASSESSMENT

The key to effective pain control is accurate assessment. Accurate assessment depends on effective communication between the nurse and patient, in particular using good listening skills and believing what patients say about their pain (Wilkinson, 1991). Whenever a patient complains of pain it is useful to use a framework of questions such as the ones in Section 7.8. It is particularly important to encourage patients to describe the pain as this can frequently indicate the cause of the pain. Muscle pain, for

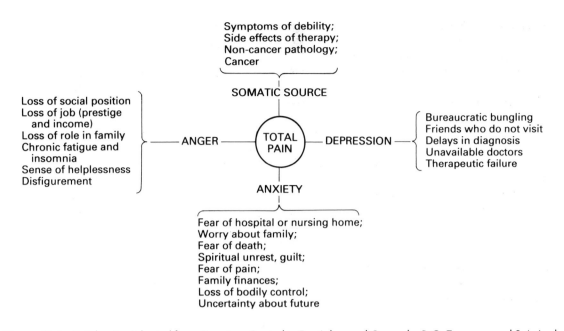

Figure 7.1 and surrounding diagram labels:

Symptoms of debility;
Side effects of therapy;
Non-cancer pathology;
Cancer

SOMATIC SOURCE

Loss of social position
Loss of job (prestige
    and income)
Loss of role in family
Chronic fatigue and
    insomnia
Sense of helplessness
Disfigurement

ANGER — TOTAL PAIN — DEPRESSION

Bureaucratic bungling
Friends who do not visit
Delays in diagnosis
Unavailable doctors
Therapeutic failure

ANXIETY

Fear of hospital or nursing home;
Worry about family;
Fear of death;
Spiritual unrest, guilt;
Fear of pain;
Family finances;
Loss of bodily control;
Uncertainty about future

Figure 7.1 Total pain. Adapted from *Symptom Control in Far Advanced Cancer* by R.G. Twycross and S.A. Lack, Pitman, London, 1983, by permission of Churchill Livingstone, Edinburgh.

example, is often described as a cramp-like pain; nerve pain is commonly described as sharp or knife-like. Fairley (1978) gives a comprehensive account of how different pains are described. Very often patients will experience more than one pain. Twycross (1984) found 80% of patients had two or more pains, while 34% of patients had four or more. It is vital that each site of pain is assessed and documented separately.

Assessment tools

In recent years there has been continued interest in the development of pain assessment tools as a means of systematically monitoring pain (Dalton, 1989). Pain assessment tools have been shown to improve pain control and aid nursing care (Berker & Hughes, 1990). There are four types of tool available for assessing and monitoring pain intensity and relief:

Categorical verbal rating scales
Categorical verbal rating scales aim to measure pain intensity and pain relief. They consist of a 4 or 5 point scale. Patients are asked to endorse the word which best describes the pain. The most usual words used are, for example, for pain intensity – none 0, mild 1, moderate 2, severe 3 or very severe/unbearable 4, or

for pain relief – none 0, slight 1, moderate 2, good 3, complete 4. Although the relative size of the differences between the words is unknown, in practice they are seen to be equal. The scales are easy and quick to complete.

Visual analogue scales
Visual analogue scales aim to measure pain intensity and relief. They consist of a straight line usually 10 cm long with extreme limits marked by a perpendicular line. Appropriate labels but no words or numbers are used between the end points. Patients are asked to mark the line with a cross at the point which represents their current pain level.

Numerical rating scales and pain thermometers
Numerical rating scales and pain thermometers are a variation of visual analogue scales used to measure pain intensity. These are scales which use numbers instead of words and are labelled 0–10 or 0–100. They are usually given verbal end points such as, 'no pain' at 0, and 'unbearable pain' at 10. Downie et al. (1978) evaluated pain rating scales and found that the 0–10 numerical scales had some advantages over the categorical verbal rating scales in terms of accuracy. Scott (1992) studied the effectiveness of using a numerical rating scale for assessing post-operative pain and

concluded that patients found the numerical rating scale easy to understand. Also, use of this scale prompted more effective pain relieving measures in acute post operative pain, which concurs with the findings of Heidrich and Perry (1982).

Questionnaires

There are several pain questionnaires available. The McGill pain questionnaire in its original or short form (Melzack, 1987) aims to assess the quality and intensity of pain, but it is difficult to score and very time consuming to administer. Other questionnaires include the diary type of monitoring tool which can be particularly useful in the community setting. Examples of diary type monitoring tools include the Royal Marsden Hospital pain chart (Walker *et al.*, 1987) or The London Hospital pain chart (Raiman, 1981). Most of the diary pain charts have been designed for completion by the patient alone or with assistance from a nurse. They focus on patients' descriptions of their pain and factors affecting its severity. Most have a body outline which enables patients to locate the sites of their pain. The pain intensity at each site is monitored using a numerical scale, usually of 0–5 with 5 relating to the worst pain. The scale can be used to re-assess pain at each site at regular intervals. Information regarding the medication administered and the patients' activities can also be recorded in relation to the pain being experienced. These pain questionnaires have been identified more for use with patients experiencing chronic pain rather than acute pain (Walker *et al.*, 1987; Raimen, 1981).

Monitoring pain

Acute pain needs to be monitored every hour and when opioid analgesia is increased observation should be made for adverse reactions. All analgesia in acute pain should be recorded as should other pain relieving measures such as a change of position. For chronic pain, the intensity of such pain, the route and dose of medication given, patient activity and any other comments made by the patient should be recorded by the patient and carer or nurse every two hours until pain control is achieved.

Pain assessment tools can be helpful in monitoring pain but they are not always appropriate as some patients are too weak or tired or unable to concentrate long enough to complete an assessment form, and some patients just do not want to have a constant two hourly reminder of how much pain they are experiencing.

7.3 GUIDANCE FOR PRACTICE – MANAGEMENT OF PAIN

The nursing management of pain begins with planning. Effective planning of care needs to involve the patient and carers as this can give them a sense of control, reduce feelings of helplessness, and help with compliance in treatment and care activities.

The pharmacological management of pain

The World Health Organisation (1990) published guidelines for the use of analgesic drugs for pain and suggested the best method of using them. The WHO framework uses an analgesic ladder with three steps. The drugs listed on the first step of the ladder are used to treat mild pain. If the pain does not respond to these drugs or is more severe, drugs from a weak opioid group on the second step of the ladder can be used. If the pain gets worse or is intolerable the drugs on the third step of the ladder may be required. The group of drugs on the third step are strong opioids and include morphine. An important point about the step ladder approach to pain control is that the patient can travel either up or down the ladder. If a patient needs to have a strong opioid to gain control of the pain it is possible that once pain control is achieved the type or strength of the analgesia may be reduced. In some instances GPs prescribe a minimum and maximum dose of an appropriate drug and develop protocols for its administration by community nurses. Following an assessment of pain the nurse is then able to decide on the correct dose within the range. The general principles of use of analgesics are shown in Table 7.3.

The decision to start using a strong opioid should be made as a logical progression and not as a last resort. It must be emphasised that not all patients with chronic pain automatically need strong opioids. If opioids are needed there is little to choose between morphine and diamorphine. The main difference lies in their stability and their solubility. Large amounts of

Table 7.3 Principles of the pharmacological management of pain.

- Pain relief depends on regular doses of analgesia and treatments should be as simple as possible, especially when treating patients in their own homes.

- A working knowledge of different analgesics is necessary.

- Dosages should be determined on an individual basis; there are no rules about the amounts of opioids required.

- Patients should never have to 'earn' their analgesia: prescribed analgesics should be given on a regular basis.

- Changing from one weak opioid to another will not achieve better pain control.

- Treatment should be administered by the oral route whenever possible, and only when a patient has persistent nausea or vomiting or is incapable of swallowing should other routes be considered.

- Opioid suppositories or continuous subcutaneous infusions are usually preferable to the intramuscular route.

- Cocktails or mixtures of drugs should not be routinely used.

- Patients starting opioid treatment should be prescribed laxatives to alleviate the side-effect of constipation.

diamorphine may be dissolved in a very small amount of liquid, which is ideal if injections become necessary.

Conversion from morphine to diamorphine

Whenever converting from morphine to diamorphine or from the oral route to the parenteral route, potency ratios need to be borne in mind. When converting oral morphine to parenteral morphine the dose must be reduced by one third. Diamorphine is 1.5 times as potent orally and 0.25 times as potent as parenteral morphine. Therefore, 10 mg of diamorphine given orally is equivalent to 15 mg of oral morphine. Both produce a duration of useful analgesia from 3 to 5 hours.

Commencing strong opioids

The easiest way of starting strong opioids is to use a simple solution of oral morphine such as morphine sulphate or oramorph. Morphine tablets to be taken 4 hourly are also available such as sevredol. The usual starting dose of oral morphine is 10–15 mg taken 4 hourly. Patients or carers can be instructed to increase the dose by 5 mg increments if the analgesia is insufficient after a few doses. Once complete pain relief has been achieved, the total daily dose of the opioid is calculated and patients can convert to 12 hourly slow release preparations of morphine, such as MST. A starting dose of 10 mg of morphine sulphate

4 hourly gives a total daily dose of 60 mg per day. Therefore, the starting dose for slow release morphine is 30 mg 12 hourly. If a patient is prescribed slow release morphine it is often useful to provide them with a bottle of morphine sulphate solution to take if break-through pain occurs as it takes time for an increased dose of slow release morphine to work. Patients should be encouraged to keep a pain diary recording the amounts of back up morphine they require over a 24 hour period so that the dosage of slow release morphine can be adjusted accordingly.

Side effects of morphine

The side effects of morphine are:

- Sedation – this usually decreases after a few doses.
- Constipation – this is inevitable and laxatives should be commenced in anticipation.
- Nausea and vomiting – some patients experience nausea during the first few days of morphine administration. If this is experienced anti-emetics need to be prescribed for a few days.
- Addiction – psychological dependence does not occur when morphine is used as an analgesic.

Alternative routes of analgesia administration

As it is not always possible to use the oral route because of the patient's condition or inability to swallow, other routes can be considered remembering that they have their individual drawbacks:

- *The sublingual route.* This route is useful for acute pain. The drugs dissolve in the mouth through the mucosa, for example, Temgesic. It is not a route usually used for those with chronic pain, particularly patients with cancer as many suffer from dry mouths with very little saliva to dissolve the tablet.
- *The rectal route.* Many drugs come in suppository form and this route may be preferred by patients if they can insert suppositories themselves, maintaining control of their medication regimen. Some patients, however, do not like this route, either because of the discomfort or the fact that this route is not acceptable culturally.
- *The parenteral route.* There are few indications for using the intravenous route for analgesia with patients suffering from chronic pain, although it can be used in acute pain management. Hickman lines may be used to deliver analgesia and are often used for children.
- *Spinal routes* for administering analgesia can be considered after systemically administered analgesia has been shown to be ineffective or have intolerable side-effects. The system for administering drugs has to be inserted surgically, and the drugs administered by a practitioner who is skilled in the technique.
- *The subcutaneous route.* Rather than giving repeated injections the use of the subcutaneous infusion via a syringe driver is preferred, especially in the community where the nurse cannot always guarantee regular times for visiting the patient. Syringe drivers are now available that enable patients to administer bolus doses of analgesia when required and these are useful for patients who need extra analgesia before or during painful procedures.

Morphine resistant pain

Morphine is not a panacea for pain relief; not all pain responds to morphine. Recent research suggests that the continuous use of high doses of morphine/ diamorphine may sometimes induce 'paradoxical pain' or an overwhelming pain syndrome in which pain ceases to be relieved or is worsened by the further administration of the drug (Morley *et al.*, 1992). It is thought that paradoxical pain arises because of abnormal metabolism of morphine wherein large amounts of morphine 3 gluconuride are formed with little or no morphine 6 gluconuride. Morley *et al.*, (1993) have illustrated that a switch from morphine to methadone may be advantageous in the treatment of pain that is uncontrolled by oral morphine. They suggest doctors should consider the switch to methadone when morphine or diamorphine has ceased to be effective. Their guidelines recommend an initial dose of methadone that is one tenth of the daily dose of morphine but not greater than 100 mg. The methadone should be given at intervals determined by the patient but not more frequently than three hourly. Patients require 3 to 8 doses per day for the first few days and then a lower fixed intake of 1 to 4 doses per day. Care needs to be taken when patients are using methadone as it has a long half life and repeated doses can lead to accumulation.

Co-analgesics

Many pains do not respond to opioids alone, and drugs known as co-analgesics are frequently given in conjunction with opioids to relieve pain.

- Non steroidal anti-inflammatory drugs (NSAID) are useful in bone pain, soft tissue infiltration and retro-peritoneal pain, e.g. flurbiprofen or naproxen. Some patients respond better to one NSAID than another. It can sometimes be beneficial to change from one if it is not effective after 1–2 weeks. If an NSAID is required via a syringe driver, Ketorolac can be used.
- Corticosteroid drugs are useful in reducing oedema and inflammation surrounding a tumour and raised inter-cranial pressure, and in nerve compression or visceral tumours. These drugs include, dexamethasone or prednisolone. Corticosteroids have a useful side effect of improving appetite and giving patients a feeling of wellbeing.
- Anticonvulsant drugs are useful for trigeminal nerve pain and can also be useful for shooting or stabbing pains, for example carbamazepine and sodium valporate.
- Anti-depressant drugs are useful for pain due to compression or destruction of nerves, for example as a result of fungating cancer of the breast. The most widely used anti-depressants as co-analgesics are amitriptyline, dothiepin and mianserin.
- Muscle relaxant drugs can be used for muscle spasms caused by pain, anxiety, disease or nerve

damage to the muscles. Diazepam may be given but can cause addiction. Baclofen is not a sedative but does have other undesirable side effects.

■ Radiotherapy is useful as a means of relieving pain in patients with advanced cancer who have developed painful bone metastases. The reduction of pain in bone metastases treated with radiotherapy appears to be achieved within 48 hours. As a result analgesics used to control the pain previously may need to then be reduced.

■ Nerve blocks are useful in localised areas or where other methods of pain relief may be contraindicated or have not worked. Injected local anaesthetic block may be effective for 12–15 hours. Phenol injections may be effective for 8–22 weeks but local anaesthetic has the advantage of being discontinued if the patient finds the loss of sensation too unpleasant.

7.4 GUIDANCE FOR PRACTICE – SYRINGE DRIVERS IN PAIN CONTROL

The syringe driver is a portable battery operated instrument allowing a continuous subcutaneous infusion of drugs over a 24 hour period. Although there is a paucity of controlled trials comparing continuous subcutaneous infusions with other routes of drug administration, a decrease of 46% in pain linear analogue scores and a 54% decrease in pain scores on the McGill pain questionnaire have been reported (Raynard, 1983). However, it is not advisable to rely on this study as the sample consisted of only six patients.

In a further study 19 patients who had received subcutaneous infusion for at least 30 days were found to have a decrease of 25% in their pain score compared with their pre-treatment score (Oliver, 1988).

The commonest problem encountered with continuous subcutaneous infusion is a reaction at the injection site, which reduces the rate of infusion. Oliver (1988) found certain medication, in particular prochlorperazine and chlorpromazine, caused this reaction. Oliver (1988) suggests it is necessary to change the injection side every few days although this is less necessary if only diamorphine is used.

Indications for use of syringe drivers

■ Inability to swallow oral medication due to:
  (a) obstruction, e.g. oral, oesophageal, intestinal;
  (b) persistent vomiting;
  (c) throat lesions;
  (d) coma.
■ Severe weakness in the terminal stage of the disease process.

The advantages of using the syringe driver in the community are many:

■ It relieves patients from the 4-hourly injection, which improves their comfort and allows them increased freedom and control.
■ A constant drug plasma level can be maintained.
■ It is unobtrusive and light to wear.
■ The site only needs to be checked and the syringe reprimed every 24 hours.
■ The patient is able to stay at home with distressing symptoms under control.

Patient education

Careful preparation of the patient is essential when changing drug medication from the oral route to the subcutaneous route, particularly as some patients feel that the syringe driver method of direct drug delivery is a last resort and that this means that their death will be imminent. One of the most important factors is to assess and acknowledge the patient's fears and concerns about this method of drug administration and give realistic reassurance as appropriate. It should be emphasised to the patient that as the drugs will be given at a constant rate this will ease the distressing symptoms for a longer period of time without having any peaks and troughs in the pain relief. When patients are receiving medication via a syringe driver it is often helpful for them to have a sheet of information to refer to when necessary.

Medication used in syringe drivers

The following list is not exhaustive, but provides an example of drugs which can be used in syringe drivers:

Analgesics
Diamorphine and morphine sulphate can be used in

whatever dose is needed for each individual patient. The advantage of diamorphine over morphine is its great solubility.

Anti-emetics
- Droperidol – often used in preference to halo-peridol.
- Metoclopramide – shown to have signs of degra-dation after one week of use. It is therefore not advisable to use it for periods longer than one week.
- Cyclizine and haloperidol. Precipitation and crystallisation within a short period of time has been demonstrated with both these anti-emetics. It is therefore advisable only to infuse these drugs in low concentrates, over a period not exceeding 24 hours.
- Hyoscine appears to remain stable over long per-iods of time in a syringe. It is therefore thought to be an ideal anti-emetic for long term, slow-running regimes. The other properties for which it can be useful are as an antispasmodic and drying agent.

- Methotrimeprazine is an extremely effective anti-emetic. Should higher concentration than 100 mg be required it should be well diluted, to lessen the risk of skin irritation.

The following medicines are not recommended for use in a subcutaneous infusion pump because they are too irritant:

- Prochlorperazine
- Chlorpromazine
- Diazepam.

Administration of drugs subcutaneously via syringe driver

There are several models of syringe drivers. The most common are the Graseby drivers MS16A and MS26. It is extremely important to check which model is being used as the drivers have different rates of delivery (Fig. 7.2).

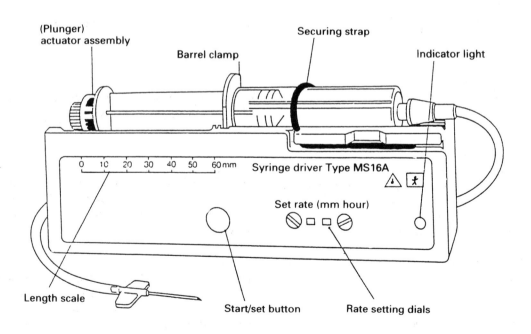

Figure 7.2 Diagram of syringe driver. Source: *The Royal Marsden Hospital Manual of Clinical Nursing Procedures* (3rd edn), Pritchard & Mallett, Blackwell Science Ltd.

Method

- Ensure that the patient is informed and consents to the procedure.
- Draw up the required solution in the syringe.
- Prime the infusion set with the solution in the syringe ensuring that no air locks are present.
- Set the calculated rate on the syringe driver.
- Slot the loaded syringe into the syringe driver securely. Ensure that the markings on the syringe are visible. Secure the rubber strap over the syringe.
- Insert the battery into the compartment in the syringe driver. The alarm will sound for a few seconds and then fade out. The battery will last for approximately 50 full syringes. The light will stop flashing 24 hours prior to it running out.
- Press the start/test button on the syringe driver. This will run for a few seconds then stop as a check that the motor safety circuits are operating.
- Go to the patient and check the patient's name against the drug prescription. (This is unnecessary in the patient's own home, but essential in residential care settings.)
- Insert the cannula into the selected site subcutaneously. Secure with transparent adhesive dressing.
  The butterfly can be situated on:
  - anterior chest wall
  - anterior aspects of upper arms or thighs
  - anterior abdominal wall
  - between scapulae.
  The following sites should be avoided:
  - lymphoedematous limbs
  - bony prominences
  - previously irradiated skin
  - near a joint.
- The syringe driver may be placed in the shoulder holster if the patient is ambulant and should be shielded from light as drugs in a syringe may degenerate when exposed to light.
- If appropriate, the start/test button can be pressed to allow a boost of the drug(s).
- Should the alarm sound, the following check should be made:
  - empty syringe
  - kinked tubing
  - blocked needle/tubing
  - jammed plunger.

Rates of administration

It is important to remember that the volume of solution in the syringe is measured in millilitres (ml). The rate of delivery from the syringe driver, however, is measured in millimetres (mm).

Different makes of syringes have different sized barrels. It is therefore important to check the length required – the ml scale against the mm scale – on the syringe driver itself, prior to commencement of each new regimen.

Daily care

- Check the site. If there is any inflammation, leakage or skin reaction change the site as this may affect the absorption and reduce the effectiveness of the drugs as well as causing discomfort. If there is no reaction change the site weekly.
- Check that the syringe driver is working and the light is flashing.
- Check that the solution remains clear.
- Check that the appropriate amount is left in the syringe. For example, when 10 ml is given over 24 hours, after 12 hours 5 ml should be left.

Weekly care

- Re-site the needle.
- Brush the screw lead with small stiff brush.

7.5 NON-PHARMACOLOGICAL METHODS OF PAIN RELIEF

Some patients do not get complete relief from conventional methods and as the complexity of pathways are becoming more readily understood the use of complementary therapies has increased as a method of achieving pain relief:

Distraction
This is the simple method of getting patients to focus on something else besides the pain, for example, listening to music or watching television. If what the patient watches or listens to is humorous this would appear to be especially effective in reducing pain (Hunt, 1993). Distraction does not make the pain go away but it tends to make the pain more bearable, i.e.

it increases pain tolerance by putting pain at the periphery of awareness.

Relaxation

This can be achieved by several techniques including yoga, simple breathing exercises or listening to a relaxation audio tape. Relaxation is not considered a pain relief measure *per se* as it does not reduce the intensity of pain. It is not a substitute for analgesia, but it can reduce the distress associated with the pain and be taught as a coping skill in response to stress.

Cutaneous stimulation

This can reduce the intensity of pain or make pain more bearable. Types of cutaneous stimulation for pain relief that are available in the home are massage, heat/cold or transcutaneous electrical nerve stimulation (TENS) machines.

Massage has been found to be particularly useful in patients with chronic pain (Simms, 1988) and good results have been achieved when a foot massage was used in conjunction with pethidine to control post operative pain (Malkin, 1994).

Aromatherapy, the use of essential oils from plants and herbs, can be used in conjunction with massage. Some oils have a stimulating and others a relaxing effect. If used as part of nursing intervention the essential oils should always be prescribed by a trained aromatherapist. There is little research that demonstrates the effectiveness of aromatherapy in reducing pain but in one study 48% of a sample of 50 patients maintained that aromatherapy massage had helped with their pain relief and 72% of the sample maintained it assisted relaxation (Wilkinson, 1994).

The application of cold is probably one of the most effective yet under used methods of relieving pain and inflammation and appears to be more effective than heat. Most nurses are taught to use heat rather than cold for pain relief, probably because the application of cold is not always acceptable to patients (McCaffery, 1990). Patients prefer heat, probably because of the initial discomfort of cold, but cooling has proved to produce more pain relief (Ramler & Roberts, 1986).

The use of TENS machines is now an accepted method of pain control. The patient can place the machine directly over or around the site of pain.

While non-pharmacological techniques for pain relief are becoming more widely used and accepted, mechanisms by which these techniques work are only partially understood and further research is necessary to quantify their value in pain control.

7.6 SUMMARY

Community nurses are regularly involved in managing patients at home who are experiencing acute or chronic pain. From the patient's perspective pain is a lived experienced and pain is whatever the patient says it is. The key to effective pain control is accurate assessment and the use of pain assessment tools has been shown to improve pain control and aid nursing care. Good pain relief depends on regular doses of analgesia, and morphine is not necessarily the panacea for all types of pain. The goal of nursing intervention should be to alleviate the patient's pain and complementary therapies may have a role to play. Nurses have a responsibility to keep up-to-date with new advances in the management of pain.

7.7 REFERENCES AND FURTHER READING

Atkinsanya, C. (1985) The use of knowledge in the management of pain: the nurse's role, *Nurse Education Today*, **5**, 6, 41–6.

Baines, M.J. (1984) Cancer pain, *Postgraduate Medical Journal*, **60**, 710, 852–7.

Berker, M. & Hughes, B. (1990) Using a tool for pain assessment, *Nursing Times*, **86**, 24, 50–52.

Bourbonnais, F. (1981) Pain assessment: development of a tool for the nurse and the patient, *Journal of Advanced Nursing*, **6**, 4, 277–82.

Camp, L.D. (1988) A comparison of nurses' recorded assessment of pain with perceptions of pain as described by cancer patients, *Cancer Nursing*, **11**, 237–43.

Cohen, F. (1980) Post surgical pain relief: patients' status and nurses medication choices, *Pain*, **9**, 265–74.

Cogan, R., Cogan, D., Waltz, W. & McCue, M. (1987) Effects of laughter and relaxation on discomfort thresholds, *Journal of Behavioural Medicine*, **3**, 139–44.

Dalton, J.A. (1989) Nurses' perception of their pain assessment skills, pain management practices and attitudes towards pain, *Oncology Nursing Forum*, **16**, 2, 225–31.

Donovan, M.I. (1985) Nursing assessment of cancer pain, *Seminars in Oncology Nursing*, **1**, 109–16.

Donovan, M.I., Dillon, P. & McGuire, L. (1987) Incidence and characteristics in a sample of medical-surgical inpatients, *Pain*, **30**, 69–78.

Downie, W.W., Leatham, P.A., Rhind, V.A., Wright, V., Branco, J. & Anderson, J.A. (1978) Studies with pain rating scales, *Annals of Rheumatic Diseases*, **37**, 4, 378–81.

Fairley, P. (1978) *The Conquest of Pain* Michael Joseph, London.

Graflam, S. (1981) Congruence of nurse–patients' expectations regarding nursing intervention in pain, *Nursing Leadership*, **4**, 2, 12–15.

Griffin, J. (1991) *Dying with Dignity* Office of Health Economics, London

Griffiths, J. & Luker, K. (1994) Community nurse attitudes to the clinical nurse specialist, *Nursing Times*, **90**, 17, 39–42.

Hanks, G.W. (1983) Management of symptoms in advanced cancer, *Update*, **26**, 1691–1702.

Heidrich, G. & Perry, S. (1982) Helping the patient in pain. *American Journal of Nursing*, **2**, 1828–38.

Hunt, A. (1993) Humour as a nursing intervention, *Cancer Nursing*, **16**, 134–9.

Latham, J. (1991) *Pain Control* second edition. Lisa Sainsbury Foundation, London.

McCaffery, M. (1983) *Nursing Management of the Patient with Pain* Lippincott Company, Philadelphia.

McCaffery, M. (1990) Nursing approaches to non-pharmacological pain control, *International Journal of Nursing Studies*, **27**, 1, 1–5

Malkin, K. (1994) The use of massage in clinical practice, *British Journal of Nursing*, 3(6), 292–4.

Melzack, R. & Wall, P. (1965) Pain mechanisms; a new theory, *Science*, **150**, 971–9.

Melzack, R. & Wall, P. (1988) *The Challenge of Pain*. Penguin, Harmondsworth.

Melzack, R. (1987) Short-form McGill questionnaire, *Pain*, **30**, 191–7.

Merskey, H. (1986) Classification of chronic pain: descriptions of chronic pain syndromes and definitions of pain terms, *Pain*, 3, Supplement S-S225.

Morley, J.S., Miles, J.B., Wells, J.C. & Bowsher, D. (1992) Paradoxical pain, *The Lancet*, **340**, 1045.

Morley, J.S., Watt, J.W.G., Wells, J.C. & Miles, J.B. (1993) Methadone in pain uncontrolled by morphine, *The Lancet*, **342**, 1243.

Oliver, D.J. (1988) Syringe drivers in palliative care: a review, *Palliative Medicine*, **2**, 21–6.

Ramler, D. & Roberts, J. (1986) A comparison of cold and warm sitz baths for relief of post partum perinial pain. *Journal of Obstetrics, Gynaecological, Neonatal Nurse*, **15**, 471–4.

Raiman, J. (1981) Responding to pain, *Nursing*, 3, 1352–65.

Raynard, C. (1983) Pain and the portable syringe pump, *Nursing Times*, **79**, 26, 25–8.

Saunders, C.M. (1964) The symptomatic treatment of incurable malignant disease, *Prescribers Journal*, **4**, 68.

Scott, I. (1992) Nurses attitude to pain control and the use of pain assessment scales, *British Journal of Nursing*, **2**, 1, 11–16.

Simms, S. (1988) Complementary therapies as nursing interventions. In *Nursing Issues and Research in Terminal Care* (Ed. by J. Wilson-Barnett and J. Raiman). John Wiley, Chichester.

Twycross, R.G. (1978) Pain and analgesics *Current Medical Research and Opinion*, **5**, 7.

Twycross, R.G. (1984) Incidence of pain, *Clinics in Oncology*, **3**, 5–15.

Ventafriddav, V., Spoldie, E., Caraceni, A., Tamburini, M. & De Conno, F. (1986) The importance of subcutaneous morphine administration for cancer pain control, *The Pain Clinic*, **1**, 47–55.

Walker, V., Dicks, B. & Webb, P. (1987) Pain assessment charts in the management of chronic pain. *Palliative Medicine*, **1**, 111–16.

Wilkinson, S.M. (1991) Factors which influence how nurses communicate with cancer patients, *Journal of Advanced Nursing*, **16**, 677–88.

Wilkinson, S.M. (1994) Aromatherapy massage – does it improve the quality of life of patients with advanced cancer? Paper presented at the 8th International Conference on Cancer Nursing, Vancouver, Canada.

World Health Organisation (1986) *Cancer Pain Relief* WHO Publications, Geneva.

World Health Organisation (1990) *Cancer Pain Relief and Palliative Care*. WHO Publications, Geneva.

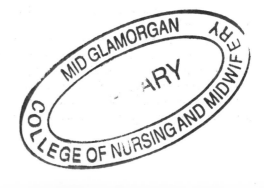

7.8 APPENDIX: PAIN ASSESSMENT QUESTIONS

Pain Assessment Questions

1. Time (Past)
 	
   a) When did the pain begin? (Hours, Weeks, Years)
 	
   b) What were you doing when it started?

2. Time (Present)
 	
   a) When do you get the pain? (Now, Daily, Weekly)
   b) During the day?
   c) At night? (How often)
   d) On movement, standing, walking bending?
   e) Is there a pattern to your pain, or is it worse at any particular time?

3. Location
 	
   a) Where is the pain?
 	
   b) Does it remain in one place or move, if so where and when?

4. Nature   a) Describe what your pain feels like (ie. burning, shooting, dull, etc.)

5. Coping
 	
   a) Is there anything which helps your pain?
   b) Is there anything you do that you find helps with the pain?

6. Effect
 	
   a) Does the pain affect your activities,
       – at home?
       – at work?
       – socially?
       – relationships (sexuality if relevant)?

7. Emotion
 	
   a) Does your pain change if you are feeling low, worried or tense?
   b) Does your pain change if you are occupied?
   c) Does your pain change if you are relaxing or enjoying yourself?

8. Treatment
 	
   a) Have you had any treatment that has had an effect on your pain?
       – medication, pain killers, others?
       – surgical treatment?
       – nerve block?
       – physiotherapy, heat massage, exercise?
       – any others such as acupuncture, relaxation therapy?

8

Promotion of Continence
Sonia Stott

Continence problems are very common and incontinence is often a source of misery for sufferers. Its unpleasant and distressing symptoms may have profound physical, psychological and social implications for sufferers, their families and their carers, (Hertzog & Fultz, 1988).

Many sufferers are reluctant to discuss their continence problem with health professionals and many believe that incontinence is an inevitable and irremediable part of the ageing process (Mitteness, 1990). However, it must be remembered that incontinence is not a disease, nor an inevitable consequence of ageing. It is a symptom rather than a diagnosis; it is never normal and is often remediable (Josephs, 1983).

In financial terms the cost of incontinence is enormous and increasing. Some £50 million per annum is spent by the NHS on pads and appliances and more than £18 million worth of appliances were provided on prescription in 1989 (Sanderson, 1991). Community nurses can play a central role in the promotion of continence.

A comprehensive nursing assessment is the primary factor in helping someone with continence problems. The assessment should be holistic, considering the physical, psychological and social needs of each individual and their influence on the problem. Information gathered at the assessment:

- helps to determine the cause of the problem;
- helps the nurse to eliminate treatable causes;
- is the basis for the plan of care;
- acts as a baseline against which progress can be evaluated

The assessment involves:

- Taking a history
- Physical examination
- Continence charting
- Clinical investigations

A continence checklist (Section 8.9) can be a useful tool for recording information obtained from the assessment. The checklist can help to ensure that all relevant areas have been covered and recorded in an accurate and systematic manner.

The assessment is best carried out in a relaxed and private atmosphere, preferably the sufferer's home. Individuals should be encouraged to talk about their continence problems in the way they see them, using their own words.

Asking the individual what they see as the main problem can be a useful starting point. But the nurse should not be surprised if there is a reluctance to admit to a problem, or if the sufferer's perception of the problems differs from the nurse's (Hafner et al., 1977). The main carer may be able to provide some of the information required to complete the assessment.

8.2 CONTROL OF MICTURITION

In infancy voiding is controlled by a simple sacral reflex arc between the bladder and the spinal cord (Fig. 8.1). As the nervous system matures and with

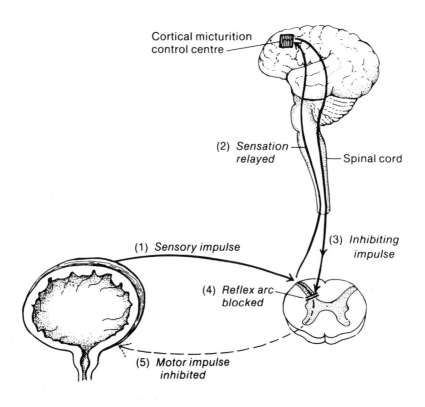

Figure 8.1   The sacral reflex arc. Source: *Nursing for Continence* by Christine Norton, courtesy of Beaconsfield Publishers Ltd.

socialisation (toilet training) we learn to appreciate the sensation of the bladder filling. Being able to recognise this sensation means that, with practice, we can override the reflex arc (Fig. 8.2).

Bladder filling causes sensory impulses to be relayed to the cerebral cortex, where voluntary control of micturition is exerted. Motor impulses which override the sacral reflex arc are relayed back down the spinal cord, delaying micturition. When an appropriate time and place are available, the cerebral inhibition is removed and micturition occurs.

Urinary incontinence

Urinary incontinence can affect anyone. Some three million people in the UK are believed to suffer from the problem (see Tables 8.1 and 8.2) (Norton, 1986). One study demonstrated that the incidence of urinary incontinence was more common in females under the age of 65 years, and that the difference tended to

equalise in the older age groups (Thomas *et al.*, 1980). The same study suggested that only a small minority ever actively seek help.

A major factor in dealing with urinary incontinence may be the negative attitudes of health professionals, which may inhibit their active involvement (Well & Brink, 1981). Effective care of the incontinent individual relies on nurses having specific research based knowledge, a broad range of up to date skills and strongly positive rehabilitative attitudes (Kings Fund, 1983).

Causes of urinary incontinence

Urinary incontinence usually results from a complex interaction of factors. Norton (1986) has divided these factors into three broad categories:

■ Physiological bladder dysfunction, including genuine stress incontinence, detrusor instability, outflow obstruction and atonic bladder.

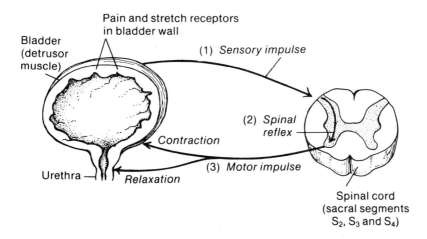

Figure 8.2 Inhibition of the sacral reflex arc. Source: *Nursing for Continence* by Christine Norton, courtesy of Beaconsfield Publishers Ltd.

Table 8.1 Prevalence of regular urinary incontinence (regular equals twice or more per month). Source: *Nursing for Continence* by Christine Norton, courtesy of Beaconsfield Publishers Ltd.

| | Age (years) | |
	15–64	65 +
Male	1.6%	6.9%
Female	8.5%	11.6%

Table 8.2 Prevalence of recognised urinary incontinence (recognised equals known to be incontinent by health, social or voluntary services). Source: *Nursing for Continence* by Christine Norton, courtesy of Beaconsfield Publishers Ltd.

| | Age (years) | |
	15–64	65 +
Male	0.1%	1.3%
Female	0.2%	2.5%

- External factors influencing bladder dysfunction, such as urinary tract infection, faecal impaction, drug therapy and endocrine disorder.
- Factors affecting the ability to cope with the bladder, such as immobility, the environment, emotional and psychological factors and the influence of carers.

8.3 GUIDANCE FOR PRACTICE – ASSESSMENT OF CONTINENCE

Determining which urinary symptoms the individual is complaining of will help to highlight bladder dys-

function. Common urinary symptoms are defined in Table 8.3.

Voiding difficulties should also be identified. These may include:

- Hesitancy
- Poor stream
- Straining
- Manual expression
- Post micturition dribble

Symptoms of voiding difficulties are usually the result of an obstructed or hypotonic bladder.

History of urinary incontinence

The nurse should establish:

Table 8.3 Common urinary symptoms.

Frequency	Most people pass urine three to four hourly, four to seven times a day. Seven or more times is usually regarded as 'frequent'.
Urgency	Having to rush to pass urine. If a toilet is not easily accessible 'urge incontinence' may occur.
Stress incontinence	Leakage of urine on physical exertion, e.g. laughing, coughing or bending.
Passive incontinence	Wetting at rest, without any coincident activity or sensation.
Nocturia	The number of times a person is awakened at night by bladder sensation.
Nocturnal enuresis	Wetting the bed whilst asleep.

- when the problem began;
- whether this was associated with any illness or event;
- what makes the problem worse;
- how often incontinent episodes occur;
- the actual volume of leakage;
- whether the problem is getting worse, static or improving.

In order to determine how leakage is dealt with and how effective any incontinence aids which may be in use are the nurse should assess:

- medical and surgical history including any gynaecological, urological, neurological disorder or surgery;
- obstetric history including number and weight of babies, type of delivery, length of labour;
- current medication, especially drugs which precipitate or exacerbate incontinence;
- usual bowel habit;
- mobility and dexterity;
- personal hygiene;
- psychological and sexual implications of the problem;
- social network, e.g. identify who provides care and the implications of incontinence for the carers;
- environmental factors – location of toilet facilities, obstacles affecting the individual's ability to cope with incontinence.

Physical examination

This should include:

- Abdominal palpation for evidence of distended

bladder which may indicate urinary retention, bladder stone or tumour.
- Vulval and vaginal examination of women for skin problems, signs of prolapse, atrophic changes, discharge and to enable estimation of pelvic floor contraction.
- Rectal examination to look for laxity of anal sphincters, prostatic enlargement, constipation and impaction.
- Neurological examination to look for evidence of stroke, diabetic neuropathy, multiple sclerosis, Parkinson's disease, etc.
- Routine urine testing – mid stream specimen of urine and residual urine if voiding problems are suspected.

Many community nurses will have developed the skills necessary for a basic physical examination which should elicit much of the information required. Further physical examination by a doctor may be necessary in some cases.

Continence charting

Recording of the individual's micturition pattern on a chart is an important aspect of the assessment. It helps to define a baseline for the problem and is used to monitor and evaluate the effectiveness of the plan of care. An accurate record of the individual's micturition pattern, episodes of incontinence, urinary output and fluid intake should be kept for between 4 and 7 days (Kennedy, 1992).

Clinical investigations

Further investigations are often required if the assessment has failed to identify the cause of incontinence or if a plan of treatment has failed to achieve continence (Cardozo, 1985).

Urodynamic studies (the study of pressure flow relationships in the lower urinary tract) may then be necessary. Basic urodynamic studies include measuring the urinary flow rate, cytometry, the measurement of detrusor pressure during controlled bladder filling and subsequent voiding and urethral pressure profile. A GP referral is usually required for such studies.

Details obtained from the continence assessment will often provide the nurse with all the information needed to identify the most likely bladder dysfunction, the factors affecting it and anything which influences the individual's ability to cope with it. It should then be possible to determine whether the overall aim of nursing treatment is to restore urinary continence, or to manage and contain incontinence (see Section 8.9).

8.4 GUIDANCE FOR PRACTICE – RESTORATION OF CONTINENCE

- Set realistic aims in conjunction with the sufferer, based on the assessment and investigations.
- Recognise that the success of any programme relies on the compliance of the sufferer and the suitability of the environment.
- Be aware of the limits of the sufferer's knowledge and expertise.

A number of interventions may be considered:

- Bladder retraining
- Toileting regimens
- Pelvic floor re-education
- Treatment of underlying disorders
- Treating constipation and promoting normal bowel function
- Advising on adequate and appropriate fluid intake
- Drug therapy
- Optimising the environment
- Clean intermittent catheterisation

Bladder retraining

Bladder retraining is aimed at treating the symptoms of frequency, urgency and urge incontinence associated with detrusor instability in order to restore a more normal or improved voiding pattern. This is achieved by gradually increasing the times between voiding.

Studies have shown that detrusor instability can be cured or much improved by a comprehensive bladder retraining programme (Jarvis, 1981). Patients usually undergo a bladder retraining programme at home, but may be admitted to hospital for this purpose.

Detrusor instability is a condition caused by uninhibited contractions which allow the bladder pressure to exceed the urethral pressure. Often patients with this condition need to rush to the toilet very frequently. Their urge to pass urine is strong and very uncomfortable. The cause of detrusor instability is often unknown (idiopathic), but may be secondary to an upper neurone lesion such as multiple sclerosis, when it is known as 'detrusor hyperreflexia' (Cardozo 1991). Similar symptoms may occur due to increased sensitivity of the bladder (sensory urge incontinence) and urodynamic investigation is necessary to aid diagnosis.

Retraining commences by establishing a baseline of frequency of micturition and incontinence charting. This enables an individual regimen to be devised.

Individuals are instructed to pass urine at set times and attempt to suppress the initial sensation of the need to pass urine. The intervals between voiding are gradually increased in an effort to reach a target three to four hour voiding pattern. The increase in time between voiding will vary from patient to patient. Much depends upon the severity of the symptoms, the motivation of the sufferer and the support available to them (Pengally & Booth, 1980). The patient is instructed to pass urine as necessary at night. Nocturia often improves as daytime voiding returns to normal.

Anticholinergic drugs may be prescribed in conjunction with a bladder retraining programme (Frewan, 1978). The drug action is to block reflex contractions of the bladder and increase urethral resistance. Encouraging the patient to carry out pelvic floor exercises (see Section 8.10), to help to inhibit the unstable contractions, may also help.

Toileting regimens

Habit retraining is a method based on the individual's usual voiding pattern. This pattern, and the occurrence of episodes of incontinence are determined by charting. A toileting programme is set, based on anticipated incontinent episodes. This typically involves the individual using the toilet just before the times when incontinence is likely to occur. As continence is achieved the intervals between toileting may be increased, which may retrain the bladder of some individuals.

Timed voiding involves taking the patient to the toilet at regular intervals (e.g. every two to four hours or before or after meals and drinks). This type of regimen ignores the individual's normal voiding pattern, so at best it will prevent some incontinent episodes; it cannot restore patients to independent continence.

Pelvic floor re-education

Pelvic floor weakness is a common cause of incontinence in women (Stanton, 1986). This condition leads to loss of urine when the intra-abdominal pressure rises, as may occur during coughing or sneezing. When there are no other symptoms, the condition is termed stress incontinence. The term genuine stress incontinence applies only when stress incontinence has been diagnosed objectively by urodynamic investigation.

Childbirth, obstetric trauma, obesity, chronic cough, lowering of oestrogen levels and straining at stool are all factors which can affect the pelvic floor muscles. Pelvic floor weakness can lead to prolapse of pelvic organs and an incompetent bladder neck sphincter mechanism.

Assessment of pelvic floor contractibility is essential before any pelvic floor exercise programme is commenced (Laycock, 1992). A physiotherapist or continence advisor who has developed expertise in this area is the best person to assess pelvic floor function and devise an appropriate exercise programme. A variety of instruction leaflets designed to advise on simple pelvic floor re-education exercises are available (see Section 8.10).

Pelvic floor exercises are the initial treatment where there is slight or moderate urine loss. The use of weighted vaginal cones, electrical stimulation, biofeedback and interferential therapy are other methods commonly employed by physiotherapists and continence advisors to assist in the re-education of pelvic floor muscle. When stress incontinence is not improved by conservative treatment, surgery may be necessary.

Treatment of underlying disorders

Many disorders exert an affect on urinary incontinence:

Severe urinary tract infection

This can result in acute frequency of micturition, urgency, pain, disturbed bladder sensation and transient incontinence. Culture and sensitivity of urine should enable the appropriate antibiotics to be prescribed. A target fluid intake should be set and monitored and analgesia given for pain. If infection occurs frequently, further investigations are necessary to identify the underlying cause.

Oestrogen deficiency

This can result in atrophic vaginitis, urethritis and trigonitis with associated symptoms of frequency, urgency and dysuria, resembling cystitis. Oestrogen deficiency is easily detected by the red, inflamed and dry appearance of vulva and vagina. Treatment is oestrogen replacement via vaginal pessaries or creams or orally.

Thyroid imbalance

This can aggravate overactive and underactive bladders, and pituitary disorders may result in excessive urine production (polyuria). Incapacitated individuals may be unable to cope with the large volumes of urine and the frequent need to void. Incontinence may occur as a result. Treatment is aimed at correcting the endocrine disorder.

Unstable diabetes mellitus

This may precipitate urinary incontinence as a result of producing large urine volumes. Glycosuria may encourage urinary tract infection.

Ensuring normal bowel function

An impacted bowel may affect the individual's urinary continence by compressing the bladder and urethra. This leads to outflow obstruction, retention of urine and overflow (Brocklehurst, 1985). Ensuring normal bowel function will eliminate the problem. The management of constipation and faecal impaction is discussed in Section 8.5.

Maintaining adequate fluid intake

Patients often restrict fluid intake in an attempt to control incontinence. Extreme fluid restriction results in dehydration, electrolyte imbalance and confusion. The incontinent patient should be aware of the need to drink normally, and may need advice on the types of fluids which should be avoided as they may stimulate the bladder, such as drinks containing caffeine or alcohol.

Drug therapy

Few drugs are effective in the treatment of urinary incontinence. Anticholinergics such as oxybutinin, imipramine and propantheline are often used in the treatment of detrusor instability in conjunction with a bladder retraining programme. Some patients are unable to tolerate the unpleasant side effects of the drugs such as dry mouth, nausea, constipation and blurred vision. The anti-diuretic drug desmopressin reduces the amount of urine produced overnight to a level which the bladder can manage, and can be an effective method of treating nocturnal enuresis.

Optimising the environment

Urinary incontinence may be precipitated or accentuated because the individual has difficulty in gaining access to an appropriate place to void. Relatively simple measures such as providing an appropriate walking aid, correcting the height of beds and chairs, and making toileting facilities more easily accessible help to optimise the environment in which the patient can cope with bladder and bowel function.

It may be that these measures are not sufficient for some individuals. Alternatives to a toilet are available and should be considered. These alternatives include the commode or chemical toilet or any one of the variety of hand held male and female urinals available. The Continence Foundation produces an up-to-date *Directory of Aids to Toileting* which provides details of suppliers and approximate prices of items available in the UK.

Clean intermittent self catheterisation (CISC)

Clean intermittent self catheterisation (CISC) is often the most effective method of managing incomplete bladder emptying. It reduces infection hazards and greatly improves the lives of many patients with disorders of micturition (Lapides *et al.*, 1972). Dribbling incontinence, voiding small amounts of urine at frequent intervals, leaking urine on physical exertion, difficulty in initiating micturition and recurrent urinary tract infections are often symptoms of incomplete bladder emptying.

When there is a persistent residual urine of more than 100 ml patients should be taught the technique of emptying their bladders with a catheter at regular intervals. CISC is a simple technique to teach. The nurse needs an understanding of bladder dysfunction and a knowledge of normal voiding patterns for it to be a safe and satisfactory practice (Winder, 1992). Principles and guidelines for CISC can be found in the Royal Marsden Hospital's manual of clinical nursing procedures (Pritchard & Mallett, 1992).

8.5 GUIDANCE FOR PRACTICE – FAECAL INCONTINENCE

Faecal incontinence is often embarrassing and distressing for suffers, resulting in humiliation and far reaching restriction of lifestyle, physical and social activities, (Lieberman, 1984). It is a problem which is often concealed for long periods or may be described by the sufferer as diarrhoea. Faecal incontinence can be defined as uncontrolled passage of stool through the rectum and is usually classified (Henry & Swash, 1985) as:

- Major incontinence – deficient control of stool of normal consistency, or
- Minor incontinence – a disorder in which there is partial soiling or occasional incontinence due to flatus or loose watery stools.

Maintenance of normal anal continence is a complex process which depends on appropriate stool consistency and volume, rectal capacity and compliance, intact sensory function and normal sphincteric function.

The causes of faecal incontinence are often classified under four main headings (Parks, 1986):

- Severe diarrhoea
- Physiological disturbance
- Neurological disorder
- Ano-rectal incontinence.

Assessment of faecal incontinence

A comprehensive nursing assessment is the primary factor in helping someone with continence problems. The assessment of faecal incontinence has much in common with the assessment of urinary incontinence. The nurse should establish in detail:

- when the problem began;
- whether this was associated with any illness or event;
- whether it is associated with impaired mobility or dexterity;
- how often incontinence occurs;
- what makes the problem worse;
- what the lost bowel content is like (e.g. consistency, amount, colour, odour, presence of blood or mucus);
- the individual's usual bowel habit (before the problem started);
- whether the individual can differentiate between solid stool, liquid stool and flatus;
- whether the individual experiences a sensation of defaecation or urgency or lacks sensation;
- whether faecal leaking occurs when coughing or bending;
- dietary and fluid intake;
- how leakage is dealt with and how effective any incontinence aids which may be in use are;
- whether the problem is worsening, static or improving;
- any relevant details of past medical, surgical and obstetric history;
- whether laxatives or constipating agents are being taken.

A patient diary, designed to record bowel habit and episodes of incontinence, can be a valuable aid in completing the overall assessment of faecal incontinence.

Physical examination

A physical examination should be carried out. This should include an assessment of the general health and mobility of the patient and rectal examination. Rectal examination should be carried out by the community nurse to exclude faecal impaction, and to look for evidence of soiling, rectal prolapse, skin excoriation, haemorrhoids and anal fissure. A more detailed rectal examination may need to be performed by a doctor.

Further investigations

These may be required if the assessment has failed to

identify the cause or when treatment has failed to achieve continence.

Treatment and management of faecal incontinence

Severe diarrhoea

Episodes of sudden, explosive diarrhoea may result in faecal incontinence. Disorders which commonly result in severe diarrhoea are inflammatory bowel disease, villous papilloma, carcinoma of the rectum, and bowel infections. Severe diarrhoea may be drug induced or result from exposure to radiation (e.g. radiotherapy). Individuals with a pelvic floor defect, impaired mobility or diminished sensation and awareness will be more susceptible to faecal incontinence after severe diarrhoea, (Barrett & Kiff, 1992).

Intervention is aimed at treating the cause of the diarrhoea and controlling symptoms. Surgical measures may be indicated where there is severe inflammatory bowel disease or cancer; anti-diarrhoeal agents may be prescribed in order to alter stool consistency.

Physiological disturbance

Severe constipation and faecal impaction are common in elderly and infirm people, particularly those who are living in nursing homes (Tobon & Brocklehurst, 1986). They also occur in young patients with delayed colonic transit and defaecatory abnormalities. The plan of care aims to promote regular, easy defaecation.

Manual evacuation of faeces may be necessary initially to remove the impacted matter. This should be followed with daily enemas and oral laxatives such as senna until the bowel is clear. Regular laxatives may be required to maintain a normal bowel habit.

Implementing a regular toileting regimen will often help to establish a normal bowel habit. The individual should be encouraged to use the toilet after meals, since food stimulates gastro-colic reflex action. It may be necessary to increase the fibre content of the individual's diet. However fibre is not always well tolerated and any change to the diet should always be gradual.

Improving mobility, adaptations to the home, review of medication that may have a constipating effect and controlling pain are all factors to be considered in promoting a regular bowel habit.

Neurological disorders

Any neurological disorder which can affect the direct

sensation or voluntary control of bowel function may result in faecal incontinence. This might include conditions such as paraplegia, multiple sclerosis, dementia, stroke, cauda equina syndrome and diabetic neuropathy.

If there is indirect indication of a full rectum and impending defaecation, e.g. sweating, flushing or tachycardia, stimulation to the rectum, either with a finger or anal dilator, may result in a bowel action. An alternative treatment involves inducing constipation with codeine phosphate or a similar drug and then emptying the bowel two to three times a week with enemas or suppositories.

Ano-rectal incontinence

Ano-rectal incontinence can result from congenital abnormalities, prolonged or traumatic childbirth, direct trauma (for example, following a road traffic accident or anal surgery), or from constant straining to pass stool. The resulting weakness of the pelvic floor muscles may result in the flap valve mechanism vital to continence being lost and rectal prolapse. Surgery is usually necessary to restore the ano–rectal angle and repair the prolapse.

Other factors which may precipitate faecal incontinence include impaired ability to communicate and psychological problems, such as depression or behaviourial disturbance. Admission to hospital or other residential care establishments, associated changes in diet, routine and environment can initiate or exacerbate the problem.

Problems can often be ameliorated through relatively simple measures such as:

- adaptations to the environment which facilitate access to the toilet;
- promoting regular toileting;
- implementation of a behaviour programme;
- improving the individual's mobility;
- reviewing medication which may have a constipating or other deleterious effect;
- controlling pain associated with defaecation.

8.6 GUIDANCE FOR PRACTICE – CONTINENCE AIDS AND APPLIANCES

A wide range of aids and appliances is currently available for patients in whom urinary or faecal incontinence proves intractable. Providing incontinence aids should rarely be the first course of action considered by the community nurse. Selection of the aid will also depend on the type, volume and frequency of urinary or faecal leakage. Gender, mobility, dexterity and eyesight and the help and care available, also sexuality should be considered.

Products available

Re-usable bodyworn pants

The re-usable bodyworn pant, e.g. the Kylie pant, provides an effective alternative to disposable pads for both males and females with light incontinence. A hydrophobic inner layer separates urine from the wearer. It is then absorbed and isolated by an outer rayon layer. This prevents the spread of urine ensuring that both the patient and the pants remain dry and comfortable.

Dribble pouch

A dribble pouch is a small disposable pouch usually made from the same absorbent material as a disposable pad and designed to fit over the penis for slight dribbling incontinence. An integral adhesive strip enables the pouch to be worn with normal well fitting underwear or with stretch net pants.

Disposable pads

Disposable underpads or bed pads are comprised of multiple layers of cellulose wadding with very little absorbency capacity or a more absorbent wood fluff pulp. They are usually faced with a water permeable non-woven coverstock and backed with polyethylene. More recent designs incorporate a cotton layer or rayon linters between coverstock and wadding while others include a superabsorber. The underpads come in a variety of lengths, thicknesses and widths, and may be sealed on two or four sides.

Disposable underpads should only be used for faecal incontinence or slight urinary leakage in bed, or as a back up in case a bodyworn pad leaks in bed. A discouraging factor as shown by trialists, is the wide misuse of this product (Ramsbottom, 1982).

Re-usable pads

Re-usable (washable) bedpads offer a much more acceptable method of protection for patients with nocturnal enuresis. These are designed to keep the urine away from the skin, keeping the patient dry. Most re-usable pads have a combined rayon and polyester absorbent layer with a hydrophobic brushed polyester facing allowing the urine to be quickly dispersed through to the middle layer where it will not flow back. The patient should lie directly on the bedsheet without nightclothes below the waist. This is not an appropriate method of containment for faecal incontinence.

Consideration should be made of the washing and drying facilities available when assessing the patient for this product, together with any help which may be available as these products become very heavy when very wet.

Penile sheaths

The penile sheath system is used with a urinary drainage bag and is suitable for men with moderate to severe urinary incontinence. It is suitable for day and night time use, and by both the ambulant and non-ambulant individual.

Penile sheaths are not suitable for men who have a retracted penis as they are unlikely to stay on. Patients with faecal incontinence are unlikely to benefit and sheaths are not advised for any patient who is likely to pull them off.

Penile sheaths are made of thin latex and designed to fit closely over the shaft of the penis. The more commonly used sheaths are kept in place by a skin adhesive. A one piece system is available in which the skin adhesive is incorporated into the inner side of the sheath which adheres to the shaft of the penis as it is unrolled. A two piece self-adhesive system has a separate double sided adhesive strip which is applied around the base of the penis and the sheath then applied over the top.

Some patients still prefer using a sheath with an external foam, velcro and elastic or latex strap fixative, which keeps the sheath in place by applying pressure around its outside.

Careful assessment for the correct size and type of sheath to suit the patient is important. The assistance of a relative or carer may be required for those who are unable to apply the sheaths themselves. Sheaths should be changed every 24 hours. Particular attention should be paid to hygiene and the skin observed for soreness or allergy.

Male bodyworn appliances

A variety of bodyworn appliances is available. These are usually semi-rigid latex cones held in place over the penis with the aid of belts and straps and connected up to a urinary drainage bag.

A pubic pressure urinal can prove very effective when a patient has a retracted penis. This aid incorporates a semi-rigid pubic pressure flange which pushes the penis forward, counteracting the tendency for retraction.

The effectiveness of an appliance depends upon a snug, comfortable fit and a downhill flow of urine at all times. They are usually fitted by a specialist surgical appliance fitter.

Patients who are heavily incontinent at night will need some method of bed protection. A wide range of products are available which can supplement the disposable and re-usable bed pad protection aids described earlier. For example, mattress covers (to fit double and single beds), duvet and pillow covers and draw sheets are available in a variety of materials such as plastic, PVC, or other water repellent fabric. To prevent odours these covers need to be wiped down daily when changing bed linen.

Urinary catheters

When all other methods of containing intractable incontinence have failed, urinary catheterisation can allow the patient a more normal and dignified lifestyle. However, insertion of a catheter should only be considered following a careful appraisal of all potential advantages and disadvantages and after full discussion between the patient, community nurse, relatives and carers.

Urinary catheters are inserted via the urethra and into the bladder in order to drain urine. Catheterisation may be either intermittent or long term depending on the patient's particular problem.

Catheter materials

The type of material from which the catheter is made will influence the length of time it may remain inserted into the bladder. Teflon (PTFE) coated latex Foley catheters are the most commonly used catheters for short to medium term insertion. They are smoother than plain latex catheters which makes them more comfortable and better tolerated (Blacklock, 1986). They can, according to manufacturers' instructions, be left *in situ* for up to 28 days.

Long term Foley catheters can remain *in situ* for up to three months. The more common types are made of 100% silicone, or silicone elastomer, or hydrogel coated silicone. Foley catheters come in two lengths, standard male length (40–45 cm) and female length (20–25 cm)

Catheter size
As a general rule, the smallest size catheter which will provide adequate drainage should be selected. For adult patients:

■ Size 12–16 Ch should be used to drain clear urine, and
■ Size 16–18 Ch should be used only for urine containing debris.

Large catheters may cause urethral irritation and trauma. Bypassing and leakage may result along with discomfort and pain and increased risk of urinary tract infection (Crow *et al.*, 1986).

Balloon size
Balloon capacities range from 5 to 30 ml. The smaller sized balloon (5–10 ml) should be used for general drainage of urine. The correct amount of sterile water should be inserted as instructed by the manufacturer. Under-inflation may result in bladder distortion and deflection of the catheter tip.

Larger balloon capacities have been found to cause bladder spasm with leakage of urine and should only be put in place by experienced urological staff following urological surgery (Roe, 1992).

A Foley catheter should always be inserted using an aseptic approach. The nursing notes should record the reason for catheterisation, the date of insertion, the amount of urine drained and any abnormalities. The size, balloon capacity, batch number and expiry date of the catheter should also be recorded.

Urinary drainage systems
Most urinary drainage systems consist of a bodyworn leg bag to which a night drainage bag can be attached. This is known as the link drainage system. Bodyworn leg bags, held by straps, suspensory systems or garments come in a range of capacities from 120 ml for children and 350 to 1500 ml for adults. Larger volume drainage bags without a tap are attached to the leg bag at night and discarded in the morning. This avoids breaking the closed system which reduces the likelihood of introducing infection. Most bodyworn bags can be used for up to a week. It is important to ensure that the patient is allowed to select a urinary drainage system, which is comfortable and manageable.

Catheter care

Once the catheter has been inserted it is essential that the patient and/or carers are advised on the maintenance of the catheter and urinary drainage system.

Personal hygiene
Hand washing before and after emptying and changing the drainage bags is essential and the safe disposal of used equipment must be encouraged.

Meatal hygiene
Normal social hygiene, a daily bath or shower and cleansing with soap and water to remove the smegma ring secreted by the glands of the clitoris and glans penis is usually sufficient. Studies suggest that the application of antibacterial creams or antiseptic lotions does not influence whether bacteriauria develops (Burke *et al.*, 1981).

Fluid intake
Adequate fluid intake (4–5 pints of liquid per day) is important, particularly in patients who are prone to catheter blocking from debris and encrustation.

Constipation
Constipation may contribute to leakage and bypassing in some patients. Measures should be taken to maintain a regular bowel habit.

Bladder washouts
The value of routine bladder washouts is questionable, although they may have a part to play for patients whose catheters constantly block due to sediment in the urine and encrustation. Generally bladder washouts should be avoided due to the risk of introducing infection by disrupting the closed system.

Education of patients and carers
Studies have shown that patients do not understand

where their catheter is located nor its function (Roe & Brocklehurst, 1987). Advice given to patients is not always based on good practice, nor consistent between nurses. A basic understanding of the location and function of the catheter will help the patient and relative to avoid problems and to deal with minor problems as they arise.

It is advisable to show the patient and carers how to manage the catheter. It may also be helpful for the community nurse to observe the patient and carer undertaking catheter care procedures. A wide range of leaflets and booklets give information on the care of catheters and urinary drainage systems. These should be made available to all catheterised patients and their carers.

As in all areas of practice, nurses need to keep abreast of current research, product and practice developments. All aspects of continence promotion and management should as far as possible be based on scientific evidence.

8.7 SUMMARY

Continence problems are a source of misery and embarrassment to many sufferers. Approximately three million people in the UK are believed to be affected. Community nurses have a key role to play in the promotion of urinary and faecal continence.

A comprehensive nursing assessment helps to determine the cause of the problem and forms the base line for the care plan. Effective care of an incontinent individual relies on community nurses having a sound knowledge base, up to date skills, and a positive attitude towards rehabilitation. It is necessary to recognise that the success of any continence programme depends on the co-operation of the patient and the suitability of the environment.

A wide range of aids and appliances is available for patients with urinary and faecal incontinence. However, aids should rarely be the first choice of action considered by the community nurse. When all other methods of containing intractable urinary incontinence have failed, catheterisation should be considered, but only following a full appraisal of both the advantages and disadvantages and after full discussion with the patient, relatives or carer.

8.8 REFERENCES AND FURTHER READING

Barrett, J.A. & Kiff, E.S. (1992) Ano-rectal function in the elderly. In *Coloproctology and the Pelvic Floor* (Ed. by M.M. Henry & M. Swash) 2nd edn. Butterworth Heinemann Ltd, Oxford.

Blacklock, N.J. (1986) Catheters and urethral strictures, *British Journal of Urology*, **58**, 475–8.

Blannin, J.P. & Hobden J. (1980) The choice of catheter, *Nursing Times*, **76**, 2092–3.

Brocklehurst, J.G. (1985) The genito urinary system – the bladder. In *Textbook of Geriatric Medicine and Gerontology* (Ed. by J.G. Brocklehurst) 3rd edition. 626–47, Churchill Livingstone, Edinburgh.

Burgener, S. (1987) Justification of closed intermittent urinary catheter irrigation/instillation: a review of current research and practice, *Journal of Advanced Nursing*, **12**, 229–34.

Burke, J.P., Garibaldi, R.A., Britt, M.R., Jacobson, J.A., Conti, M. & Ailing, D.W. (1981) Prevention of catheter associated urinary tract infections, *American Journal of Medicine*, **70**, 655–8.

Cardozo, L. (1985) Urological symptoms in women, *Maternal and Child Health*, **10**, 12, 361–5.

Cardozo, L. (1991) Urinary incontinence in women: have we anything to offer? *British Medical Journal*, **303**, 1453–7.

Crow, R.A., Chapman, R.G., Roe, B.H. & Wilson, J.A. (1986) *A Study of Patients with an Indwelling Urethral Catheter and Related Nursing Practice.* Nursing Practice Unit, University of Surrey.

Frewan, W.K. (1978) An objective assessment of the unstable bladder of psychosomatic origin, *British Journal of Urology*, **50**, 246–9.

Hafner, R., Stanton, S. & Guy, J. (1977) A psychiatric study of women with urgency and urge incontinence, *British Journal of Urology*, **49**, 211–14.

Henry, M.M & Swash, M. (1985) *Coloproctology and the Pelvic Floor.* Butterworth Heinemann Ltd, Oxford.

Herzog, A.R & Fultz, N.H. (1988) Urinary incontinence in the community: management and beliefs, *Topics in Geriatric Rehabilitation*, **2**, 1–12.

Jarvis, G.J. (1981) A controlled trial of bladder drill and drug therapy in the management of detrusor instability, *British Journal of Urology*, **53**, 565–6.

Josephs, C. (1983) Urinary incontinence, *Geriatric Medicine*, **13**, 9, 650–51.

Kennedy, A.P., Brocklehurst, J.G., & Lyne, M.D.W. (1983) Factors related to the problems of long term catheterisation, *Journal of Advanced Nursing*, **8**, 3, 207–12.

Kennedy, A.P. (1992) Bladder reeducation for the promotion of continence. In *Clinical Nursing Practice – the Promotion and Management of Continence* (Ed. by B.H. Roe) Prentice Hall International (UK) Ltd.

Kings Fund (1983) *Action on Incontinence – Report of a Working Group.* Project paper No. 43. Kings Fund Publishing, London.

Lapides, J, Dionko, A.G., Silber, S.J. & Lowe, B.S. (1972) Clean intermittent catheterisation in the treatment of urine tract disease, *Journal of Urology*, **107**, 458–61.

Laycock, J. (1992) Pelvic floor re-education for the promotion of continence. In *Clinical Nursing Practice – the Promotion and Management of Continence* (Ed. by B.H. Roe). Prentice Hall International (UK) Ltd.

Lieberman, D.A. (1984) Common ano-rectal disorders, *Annals of Internal Medicine*, **101**, 837–46.

Mitteness, L.S. (1990) Knowledge and belief about urinary incontinence in adulthood and old age, *Journal of the American Geriatrics Society*, **38**, 3, 374–8.

Norton, C. (1986) The problem of incontinence. In *Nursing for Continence*. Beaconsfield Ltd, Beaconsfield, Bucks.

Norton, C. (1988) The development of continence and causes of incontinence. In *Nursing for Continence*. Beaconsfield Ltd, Beaconsfield, Bucks., **2**, 9–26.

Parks, A.G. (1986) Faecal incontinence. In *Incontinence and its Management* (Ed. by D. Mandelstam) 2nd edition Croom Helm, Kent. **4**, 79–93.

Pengally, A.W. & Booth, G.M. (1980) A prospective trial of bladder training as treatment for detrusor instability, *British Journal of Urology*, **52**, 463–6.

Pritchard, P.A. & Mallett, J. (Eds) (1993) *The Royal Marsden Hospital Manual of Clinical Nursing Procedures.* Blackwell Scientific Publications, Oxford.

Ramsbottom, F.J. (1982) The use of incontinence underpads in hospital, *Nursing Times*, 3, November, 1868–9.

Read, N.W., Harford, W.V., Schmulen, A., Read, M.G. Santa Ana, G.A. & Fordtran, J.S. (1979) A clinical study of patients with faecal incontinence and diarrhoea, *Gastroenterology*, **76**, 747–56.

Roe, B.H. & Brocklehurst, J.G. (1987) Study of patients with indwelling catheters, *Journal of Advanced Nursing*, **12**, 713–18.

Roe, B.H. (1989) Study of information given by nurses for catheter care to patients, *Journal of Advanced Nursing*. **14**, 3, 203–11.

Roe, B.H. (1992) Use of indwelling catheters. In *Clinical Nursing Practice – the Promotion and Management of Continence* (Ed. by B.H. Roe) Prentice Hall International (UK) Ltd.

Sanderson, J. (1991) *An Agenda for Action on Continence Services.* Department of Health, London.

Smith, A.R.B., Hosker, G.L. & Warrell, D.W. (1989) The role of partial deprevation of the pelvic floor in the aetiology of genito urinary prolapse and stress incontinence of urine, *British Journal of Obstetrics and Gynaecology*, **96**, 24–8.

Smith, A.R.B., Hosker, G.L. & Warrell, D.W. (1989) The role of pudendal nerve damage in the aetiology of genuine stress incontinence in women, *British Journal of Obstetrics and Gynaecology*, **96**, 29–32.

Stanton, S.L. (1986) Gynaecological aspects. In *Incontinence and its Management* (Ed. by D. Mandelstam) 2nd edition. Croom Helm, Kent.

Thomas, T.M., Plymat, K.R., Blannin, J. & Meade, T.W. (1980) Prevalence of urinary incontinence, *British Medical Journal*, **281**, 1243–5.

Tobon, G.A. & Brocklehurst, J.G. (1986) Faecal incontinence in residential homes for the elderly: prevalence, aetiology and management, *Age and Aging*, 15, 41–6.

Well, T. & Brink, C. (1981) Urinary incontinence: assets and management. In *Nursing the Aged* (Ed. by I. Burnside) McGraw-Hill, New York.

Winder, A. (1992) Intermittent self-catheterisation. In *Clinical Nursing Practice – the Promotion and Management of Continence* (Ed. by B.H. Roe) Prentice Hall International (UK) Ltd.

8.9 APPENDIX: COMMUNITY CONTINENCE ASSESSMENT CHECKLIST

Please refer to assessment guidelines where necessary

Name _____ *DOB* _____

Address _____ *GP* _____

_____ *Consultant* _____

Tel No. _____ *Assessment date* _____

Source of referral _____ *Signature of assessor* _____

Tick (√) where appropriate/ Give more details as necessary

| Type of Incontinence | | | Medical History |

	Day	Night
Urinary	☐	☐
Faecal	☐	☐

Urinary symptoms

Frequency ☐	Urgency ☐
Urge incontinence ☐	Stress ☐

Post micturition dribble ☐

Post prostatectomy dribble ☐

Nocturia ☐

Nocturnal enuresis ☐

Passive incontinence ☐

Dysuria ☐

Haematuria ☐

Voiding difficulties

| Hesitancy ☐ | Straining ☐ |
| Poor stream ☐ | Manual expression ☐ |

When did the problem start ? ☐☐☐
                           dd mm y r

No. of episodes of incontinence ☐
In 24 hours

Surgical History

Obstetric History

No. of pregnancies ☐   Menopause age ☐

Difficult deliveries _____

Large babies _____

Learning difficulties

Physical difficulties

Current medication

Degree of Incontinence

Light [ ]   Heavy [ ]
Moderate

Previous Investigations for Incontinence ?

Fluid Intake

No. of cups in 24 hours [ ]
Are fluids restricted ?

Mobility

Fully mobile [ ]   Chairbound [ ]

Mobility impaired [ ]   Bedfast [ ]

Walks with aids [ ]

Bowel habit

Normal bowel habit [ ]   Constipation [ ]

Diarrhoea [ ]   Impaction [ ]

Faecal incontinence [ ]   Regulated with [ ]
laxatives

Regulated with diet [ ]

Dexterity

Full [ ]   Limited [ ]   Poor [ ]

General Health

Type of diet _____

Overweight ? _____

Cigarettes - no. per day [ ]

Alcohol - units per week [ ]

Caffeine drinks _____

Attitude to Incontinence

Embarrassment [ ]   Anxiety [ ]

Depression [ ]   Apathy [ ]

Denial [ ]   Learned to [ ]
cope

Toileting

Can the patient get to the toilet ? [ ]

Does s/he need any help ? [ ]

In there anyone available ? [ ]

Can the patient transfer easily ? [ ]

Pattern of Incontinence

Results from _____
baseline chart _____

Toileting facilities

Toilet location _____

[ ] Chemi toilet [ ] Commode

[ ] Urinal [ ] Bedpan

Other

Environmental/circumstantial contributions to Incontinence

Products used prior to assessment

Type   Day _____   Night _____

Quantity [ ]   Day _____   Night _____

Are the products effective ? _____

Results of physical examination   *(where necessary)*

Skin problems _____   *Vaginal examination* _____

_____   _____

Rectal examination _____   *Atrophic changes* _____

_____   _____

MSSU/Urine Test _____   *Residual Urine* _____

_____   _____

Other important findings _____

Pelvic Floor Assessment

	Yes	No
Is stress incontinence demonstrated ?		

	Yes	No
Has patient ever been catheterised ?		

	Yes	No
Can patient interrupt stream ?		

Summary of problems *Type/cause/degree of incontinence*

_____

Referral

	Yes	No			Yes	No
General Practitioner				Continence adviser		

Consultant/Physiotherapist/Occupational Therapist/Social Services/Dietitian/other _____

(Please circle each professional agency referred to. Name "Other" if category used)

Nursing Management

Urine: Routine test: _____   MSSU _____

Clear impaction   _____

Continence charting   _____

Pelvic floor exercises   _____

Toilet programme   Individualised toileting [ ]   Timed voiding [ ]   Bladder retraining [ ]

Behaviour modification   _____

Intermittent catheterisation _____

Advice   *Dietary/fluid advice/hygiene/clothes adaptation*

Continence promotion aids   Commode [ ]   Bedpan [ ]   Urinal [ ]

Other _____

Incontinence management   Incontinence pads [ ]   Laundry service [ ]

Body worn appliance [ ]   Sheath system [ ]

Urethral catheter [ ]

Review date

Notes

8.10 APPENDIX: PELVIC FLOOR ESSENTIAL EXERCISES. SOURCE: *ESSENTIAL EXERCISES FOR WOMEN – PUBERTY TO MENOPAUSE AND BEYOND, M. DOLMAN & K. SIMON, COURTESY OF PROCTER & GAMBLE PATIENT CARE DIVISION.*

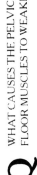

Q WHAT ARE THE PELVIC FLOOR MUSCLES?

A These muscles are most important in women, yet so often forgotten. It is the hammock-like group of muscles between your legs; attached to the pubic bone at the front and the base of the spine (coccyx) at the back. It has three openings through it, namely, anus (back passage), vagina (birth canal) and urethra (bladder outlet). Their task is to constrict and lift, to control the sphincter muscles (the muscles which close these openings).

This leaflet will explain its importance and why exercises are necessary throughout your lifetime.

Q WHAT CAUSES THE PELVIC FLOOR MUSCLES TO WEAKEN?

A When a muscle is not exercised it will weaken through lack of use. The pelvic floor muscles are no exception. The main cause is the strain and stretching in childbirth, particularly 'bearing-down' during the second stage of labour. The muscle is further stretched by babies over 8lbs in weight and with the use of forceps. Tears to this muscle or episiotomies during delivery can cause further damage. A long history of constipation problems can also weaken the pelvic floor muscles.

Q WHY SHOULD I EXERCISE THESE MUSCLES?

A This hammock-like muscle supports the three openings through it, anus, vagina and urethra. When it is weakened, it cannot support these openings effectively. The result can be leakage of urine from the bladder when you exert abdominal pressure as in coughing, laughing, jogging or keep-fit activity. Prolapses may occur through the weakened vaginal walls or even worse, bowel control may be lost.

Q HOW OFTEN SHOULD I EXERCISE THE PELVIC FLOOR MUSCLES?

A Depending on how weak the muscle is, the number of daily exercises will vary for each individual. However, aim at 50 a day and increase over a few weeks to 120 daily. Once you have 'toned up' your muscles, do enough repetitions per day to ensure that symptoms of urine leakage do not occur.

Q HOW WILL I KNOW HOW MANY EXERCISES TO DO AT A TIME?

A A weak muscle will tire if over exercised and you may experience some aching in it. If this is the case, only do a few at a time and repeat that number in several sessions a day until you have reached 50, 75, 100 or 120.

Q HOW DO I DO PELVIC FLOOR EXERCISES?

A 1. Sit comfortably with feet touching the floor, legs slightly apart. Lean forward and rest elbow on thighs. This relaxing position will ensure you do not tighten your buttocks or abdominal muscles while exercising the pelvic floor muscle.

2. Tighten and pull up the muscle around the anus, hold to the count of 3 or 4 and relax to the count of 3 or 4.

3. Now concentrate on the vagina and draw the muscle upwards and inwards and hold to the count of 3 or 4 then relax to the count of 3 or 4.

4. Repeat this drawing up and relaxing to the count of 3 or 4 with both parts of the muscle as often in an hour as you can without tiring it, that is without it aching. The total in a day should be between 50 and 120. A guideline is to do 5-10 each exercise session, gradually increasing the 'hold' times.

When you are confident that you are doing these exercises, correctly you will be able to do them whilst standing, lying or sitting. In fact you can carry out the exercises ANYTIME, ANYWHERE.

When you commence your exercise programme:

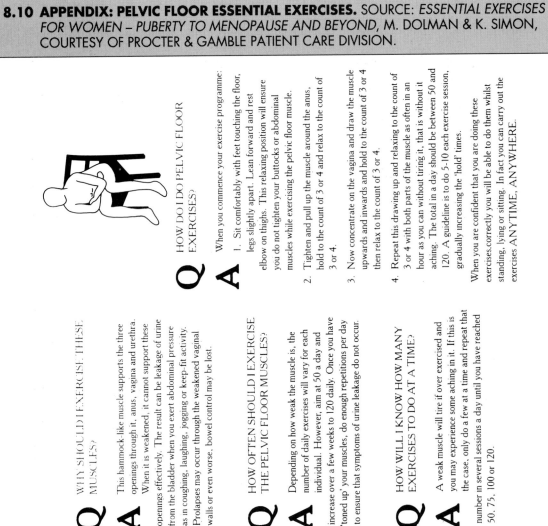

Pubic Bone   Womb   Rectum

Bladder

Pelvic floor in good condition

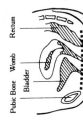

A pelvic floor that has become weakened

ESSENTIAL EXERCISES

FOR WOMEN

PUBERTY TO MENOPAUSE & BEYOND

Information leaflet on the Pelvic Floor written by professionals

Written by:

Mary Dolman BSc RGN
Clinical Nurse Specialist
East Berkshire Health Authority

Kay Simon MCSP BA(Hons)
Physiotherapist

Procter&Gamble

Procter and Gamble Ltd, Patient Care Division,
St. Nicholas Avenue, Gosforth, Newcastle upon Tyne NE99 1EE.

Q ARE THERE ALTERNATIVE PREVENTATIVE MEASURES TO THESE EXERCISES?

A No. **All women** need to maintain the muscle tone of their pelvic floor.

REMEMBER PREVENTION IS BETTER THAN CURE

It costs nothing to do these exercises, only the memory to do them daily.

Q IF I HAVE SYMPTOMS OF PELVIC FLOOR WEAKNESS WILL THESE EXERCISES HELP ME?

A Yes . . . However, you may need a more intense exercise programme. These can be individually devised for you by a Specialist nurse or physiotherapist.

Treatment available can include stimulation of the pelvic floor muscles or the use of weighted vaginal cones. For extreme cases surgery may be indicated.

Produced by:

Procter and Gamble Ltd, manufacturer of the LIC Daisy and Attends Ultra Care range of incontinence products.

For further information about LIC Daisy and Attends Ultra Care products please call FREEPHONE 0800 590555.

9

Management of Hypertension

Ann-Louise Caress and Maria Kenrick

9.1 INTRODUCTION

Raised blood pressure is a common problem throughout the industrialised world. It is estimated that 0.5% of the population of the United Kingdom have severe hypertension requiring urgent attention, 10–15% have diastolic blood pressures over 100 mmHg and require medication, and 20% have diastolic blood pressure in the 90–99 mmHg range and require systematic follow up (Hart, 1993; Bannan et al., 1987). In a general practice population of 2500 these proportions would mean 253 patients with a degree of high blood pressure.

It is widely recognised that high blood pressure is one of the risk factors for coronary heart disease and stroke, which remain the largest causes of morbidity and mortality in the United Kingdom (Anderson, 1988). The risk of coronary heart disease and stroke rises from less than 10% in those with a systolic blood pressure of 120 mmHg to almost 60% in those with a systolic reading of 200 mmHg (Bannan et al., 1987).

With the recognition of the potential for reducing morbidity and mortality through action to reduce blood pressure, and the impetus of the 1990 GP contract, increasing attention has been given to the monitoring and treatment of blood pressure. The role of the community nurse in this has been considerable, particularly with the rapid expansion in the numbers of practice nurses, who are often responsible for undertaking blood pressure screening.

9.2 AETIOLOGY OF HYPERTENSION

Since there is a wide range of blood pressure variation within a given population, defining pathological hypertension can be difficult. In the past diagnosis of hypertension was typically based on the diastolic value only. However, it is now recognised that the systolic reading can also be of significance (Beevers & Wilkins 1987; Hart, 1993), particularly in older people (Systolic Hypertension in the Elderly Programme Co-operative Research Group, 1991). It is suggested that a systolic reading of 160 mmHg or above should be considered abnormal, even if the diastolic value is below 90 mmHg.

The causes of hypertension

High blood pressure is typically divided into primary or essential hypertension and secondary hypertension, the difference between the two being that in the latter the raised blood pressure can be attributed to another disease entity whilst in essential hypertension it cannot.

High blood pressure is widely recognised as being multifactorial in origin (Beevers & Wilkins 1987; Hart, 1993). A number of contributing factors to essential hypertension have been identified:

- Stress
- Dietary factors (sodium and potassium intake; cholesterol)
- Obesity
- Alcohol consumption

- Demographic variables (sex, race, social class)
- Smoking

Secondary hypertension is associated with:

- Renal disease
- Diabetes
- Coarctation of the aorta
- Phaeochromocytoma
- Intercranial tumours
- Endocrine disorders.

The Royal College of General Practitioners (1981) also identifies a number of iatrogenic causes of hypertension:

- Oral contraceptives
- Monoamine oxidase inhibitors (MAOIs)
- Non-steroidal anti inflammatory drugs
- Sympathomimetic amines (in some decongestants and eye drops).

The symptoms of hypertension

Many patients with hypertension are asymptomatic, and the usual symptoms of high blood pressure are common to other disorders. Therefore, identifying those with hypertension can be a difficult undertaking. Known symptoms of hypertension include:

- Headache
- Fatigue
- Dyspnoea
- Dizziness
- Palpitations
- Mood disturbances
- Erectile impotence.

A number of other clinical signs may also be identifiable and evidence of any of these would be suggestive of hypertension and associated organ damage:

- Retinal haemorrhages
- ECG and/or X-ray evidence of left ventricular hypertrophy
- Proteinuria and haematuria.

Clinical signs suggestive of the presence of an underlying pathology known to give rise to hypertension may also be evident. These would include glycosuria or raised blood glucose levels suggestive of diabetes; proteinuria or haematuria (not associated with malignant hypertension) suggests renal disease. In a number of conditions such as hypokalaemia, primary aldosteronism or renal disease, alterations in blood biochemistry would be evident (Beevers & Wilkins, 1987).

9.3 CLINICAL MANAGEMENT OF HYPERTENSION

Many individuals with even markedly raised blood pressures will be asymptomatic. By contrast, many of those who receive medication for hypertension will experience unpleasant side effects (Hart, 1993; Medical Research Council, 1981). Even in the absence of medication, patients can experience anxiety and lifestyle disruption as a result of having their blood pressure treated (Beevers & Wilkins, 1987). There is some consensus as to the need for treatment of very high blood pressures. However, for lower values, there is less agreement, since the disadvantages of intervention (e.g. medication side effects, patient anxiety, need for follow up) may outweigh the benefits of reduced blood pressure.

A number of factors must be considered before treatment is commenced (Bannan et al., 1987). These include considerations about the age and sex of the patient; the presence of other cardiovascular risk factors (e.g. diabetes, smoking, obesity, family history); the extent of intervention required and its impact on available resources; and the likelihood of patient compliance. An important consideration is evidence of organ damage, which indicates a need for prompt commencement of therapy.

The British Hypertension Society guidelines (Swales et al., 1989) recommend that treatment for high blood pressure should be commenced after three consecutive readings of a diastolic blood pressure of more than 100 mmHg in a four month period, even if the patient is asymptomatic.

Non-pharmacological interventions

A number of non-pharmacological interventions have been suggested for the management of mild to moderate hypertension. These typically involve some form of behaviour modification on the part of the patient, in the form of stress reduction (lowering salt, alcohol and cholesterol intake), increasing exercise and reducing weight (Beevers & Wilkins, 1987; Department of Health and Social Security, 1984; Hart, 1993).

However, behavioural change is often difficult to accomplish and many such interventions are ineffective (Hart, 1993). Furthermore, relative to the time and lifestyle disruption to be gained, the benefits are questionable. Sodium restriction is one such intervention, where severe reduction of salt intake may be effective in lowering blood pressure, but unacceptable to patients because of its effect on the palatability of their food (Beevers & Wilkins, 1987). Where behaviour modification is indicated the community nurse has an important role in helping hypertensive patients to make informed decisions about their health.

Pharmacological interventions

Traditional medication for hypertension, consists of beta-blockers accompanied by a thiazide diuretic (Beevers & Wilkins, 1987). Recent pharmacological developments have broadened the range of available medications to include calcium antagonists such as verapamil, nifedipine, and diltiazem and angiotensin converting enzyme inhibitors enalapril and captopril.

For resistant hypertension, a combination of medications is often used. Furthermore, there are other agents which may be considered, notably direct acting vasodilators such as hydralazine and minoxidil. Alternatively diuretics (such as spironolactone or amiloride) may also be used.

Pharmacological interventions present a number of problems, the main one being medication side effects. A further problem is patient compliance. Medication non-compliance has been noted as a problem in hypertension treatment (Haynes, 1982). Furthermore, consideration must be made of co-existing morbidity, such as renal disease, heart failure, asthma and other drugs being taken by the used.

9.4 GUIDANCE FOR PRACTICE – MONITORING BLOOD PRESSURE

The Department of Health made blood pressure screening one of the health promotion targets in the 1990 GP contract, and it is estimated that more than 90% of general practices now have health promotion clinics at which routine blood pressure measurement is undertaken (Hart, 1993).

In general practices, blood pressure may be recorded either by the doctor or the nurse. There is evidence which suggests that nurses with appropriate training may actually be more reliable in recording blood pressures than doctors (Hart, 1993).

For patients in whom hypertension is identified, repeated measurements of blood pressure may be required. This can be inconvenient for patients and a drain on the resources of a practice. For these reasons, increasing use is being made of patient self-measurement of blood pressure after appropriate training (Beevers & Wilkins, 1987).

Accurate blood pressure measurement is dependent on:

- The patient
- The observer
- The equipment.

The patient

A number of physiological features can influence a patient's blood pressure, including age, sex, temperature, emotional state and any underlying morbidity (Bannan *et al.*, 1987). These should be taken into account when monitoring blood pressure.

Attention should be paid to adequate preparation of the patient before recording the blood pressure. The observer should ensure that the patient is comfortable, warm and rested. Ideally the blood pressure should not be recorded within 15 minutes of the patient having eaten or smoked. When any of these conditions cannot be met a note should be made on the blood pressure recording sheet (Bannan *et al.*, 1987).

A full bladder can have a hypertensive effect, so where an unusual reading is recorded enquiries should be made as to whether the patient needs to micturate.

The arm in which the blood pressure is to be recorded should be supported and held horizontal at the level of the fourth intercostal space (Bannan *et al.*, 1987). Failure to do either of these things can distort the reading obtained by as much as 10 mmHg. The blood pressure is typically recorded on the right arm; however, the first recording should be made on both arms. Large differences between the left and right arms (at least 20 mmHg systolic) should be noted and the measure repeated to see if the difference persists.

Prevention of venous congestion is important as this can distort a reading. Tight clothing should be removed from the limb on which the blood pressure is to be measured, but if this is not possible then it is preferable to put the sphygmomanometer cuff over a tight sleeve than to roll the sleeve up and create a tourniquet effect. If blood pressure measurements are to be repeated then adequate time between readings must be allowed to prevent venous congestion from occurring.

The observer

A number of faults and biases on the part of the observer can be sources of error in blood pressure recordings. Firstly, the observer may unconsciously bias the recording to favour a prior expectation about the patient. For example, if the patient is obese a borderline value is more likely to be labelled hypertensive than the same reading in a slimmer person (Bannan et al., 1987).

The tendency to do this is exacerbated by a second observer bias known as 'digit preference' (Hart, 1993). This is when the observer rounds up or rounds down the blood pressure reading to the nearest 5 mmHg or terminal digit. The correct procedure for recording should be to chart the actual value, which on most sphygmomanometers will be in intervals of 2 mmHg.

Incorrect eye positioning relative to the instrument can cause errors in recording. A mercury manometer must be placed so that the observer's eye is level with the meniscus of the mercury column, whilst an aneroid machine must be viewed straight on. Incorrect placement of a mercury sphygmomanometer can give rise to an erroneous reading. The machine should be placed upright on a flat surface, level with the subject's arm (Kemp et al., 1993).

Poor observer skills and undue haste in taking the recording have been identified as potential sources of error (Bannan et al., 1987; Kemp et al., 1993). For example, releasing cuff pressure too rapidly will cause the systolic value obtained to be lower than its actual value, whilst the recorded diastolic value will be higher than its actual level. Bannan et al., (1987) suggest that more attention needs to be paid to training, both in initial teaching and in terms of on-going in-service training to identify and correct poor habits (see Table 9.1, below).

Table 9.1 Procedure for recording blood pressure (after Bannan et al., 1987).

- Remove tight clothing.
- Apply bladder, ensuring snugness of fit.
- Palpate the brachial artery, then rapidly inflate the cuff to 30 mmHg above the disappearance of the pulse.
- Deflate the cuff slowly until the pulse reappears and note this point (systolic value).
- Place the diaphragm of the stethoscope over the brachial artery.
- Inflate the cuff to a point 30 mmHg above the palpated systolic value.
- Deflate the cuff at the rate of 2–3 mmHg per second.
- Note the appearance of the first sound as the systolic value.
- Note the point at which the sound disappears as the diastolic value.
- Deflate the rest of the cuff.
- Chart the measured values to the nearest 2 mmHg.
- If the reading is raised, wait for an interval and repeat the measurement.

more commonly called, is now considered to be the method of choice for monitoring glycaemic control (Walker, 1993). If undertaken properly, it is more accurate than urine testing and the technique is simple and inexpensive. The technique involves collection of a drop of capillary blood, usually from a finger (although an earlobe may be used) and placing it onto a reagent strip. The result may be read by eye or using a meter. It is possible for most patients to contribute to HBGM. Special devices are available for use with blind or visually impaired patients. HBGM is a relatively simple technique which gives patients information on which to base the day-to-day management of their treatment. The community nurse has a role in teaching patients how to use monitoring equipment.

The use of meters to interpret blood glucose values is increasingly common (Walker, 1993). Meters have the advantage of giving an accurate reading, which helps to combat errors of interpretation, visual impairment and colour blindness. A range of such products exists and the advice of a specialist diabetic nurse or the British Diabetic Association would be useful in helping patients select appropriate machinery.

10.5 GUIDANCE FOR PRACTICE – MANAGEMENT OF THE COMPLICATIONS OF DIABETES

There are a number of conditions associated with diabetes which may need to be dealt with by nurses in the community. These include:

- Hypoglycaemia
- Ketoacidosis
- Foot problems
- Surgery and medication
- Non-compliance with treatment.

In addition pregnancy can be dangerous for the woman with diabetes.

Hypoglycaemia

Hypoglycaemia is a common, distressing and poten-

tially life-threatening complication of diabetic treatment. Hypoglycaemia occurs when blood glucose falls below about 2.5 mmol/l (Watkins, 1993). It is estimated that more than 30% of diabetics on insulin experience hypoglycaemic coma at least once and approximately 3% of patients on insulin suffer frequent and incapacitating hypoglycaemia (Williams & Pickup, 1992).

The main cause of hypoglycaemia is an imbalance between the amount of hypoglycaemic agent and the exercise level and food intake of the patient. It is common at night in those on oral hypoglycaemics and these patients may become fearful of dying in their sleep. Most patients are awakened by hypoglycaemia (or by a partner who notices restlessness or sweating). A small number of patients, however, do not awaken and may progress to coma; this is particularly problematic if the patient lives alone. Other times when hypoglycaemia may occur are after:

- the commencement of therapy;
- weight loss;
- delivery of a baby;
- a missed meal;
- consumption of alcohol;
- a change in therapy.

Symptoms of hypoglycaemia are progressive and later symptoms are the result of glucose starvation in the brain. Early symptoms include:

- Tremor
- Sweating
- Hunger
- Palpitations
- Pins and needles in the lips and tongue.

Symptoms of mild brain glucose starvation (neuroglycopenia) include:

- Double vision
- Poor concentration
- Slurred speech.

Symptoms of severe neuroglycopenia include:

- Confusion
- Behaviour change (e.g. aggression)
- Unconsciousness.

It is important to note that symptom awareness

may be blunted or absent in some patients, notably older people, long standing diabetics and patients with autonomic nerve damage (Paterson, 1990; Williams & Pickup, 1992). It is therefore important that relatives and carers be taught to recognise hypoglycaemic symptoms, and particularly be advised that stubborn denial of hypoglycaemia is common and is caused by neuroglycopenia.

Prevention of hypoglycaemia involves:

■ regular monitoring of blood glucose and adjustment of carbohydrate intake;
■ increasing patient awareness of the symptoms of hypoglycaemia;
■ increasing patient awareness of precipitating factors.

For example, nocturnal hypoglycaemia can often be prevented by performance of a pre-bed blood glucose reading. Watkins (1993) suggests that if the value is below 5 mmol/l, the patient should take some additional carbohydrate before retiring.

Once hypoglycaemia has occurred, the action taken will depend upon whether or not the patient is conscious. In a conscious patient, 10–20 g of sugar should be taken orally. This may be in the form of: milk (about $\frac{1}{2}$ pint contains 10 g); a sweet drink (e.g. 60 ml Lucozade); sugar (2 teaspoons contain 10 g) or dextrose tablets (3 Dextrosol tablets contain 10 g). It is important that patients be taught to keep such agents readily available in the home, in the car, and in pockets.

Oral therapy should not be attempted in an unconscious patient. Instead treatment should be either by intramuscular injection of 1 mg of glucagon or with an intravenous bolus of glucose, e.g. 30 ml of 20% solution (Williams & Pickup, 1992).

Glucagon injection is the first line therapy for unconscious patients who are at home; the drug and appropriate equipment should be kept in a readily accessible place and relatives or carers will need instruction on how to give a glucagon injection. It is important to note that glucagon may take up to 20 minutes to work and that the patient will need to eat as soon as possible after recovery since the effect of glucagon is transient (Drury, 1986).

In patients with hypoglycaemia subsequent to taking sulphonylureas or long acting insulin, hospital admission and commencement of intravenous dextrose infusion may be necessary to correct hypogly-

caemia and prevent relapse (Drury, 1986; Williams & Pickup, 1992). Once the patient has recovered from the hypoglycaemic attack it is important to establish, if possible, precipitating factors, so that future episodes may be prevented.

Ketoacidosis

Ketoacidosis occurs as a result of a lack of insulin, which gives rise to hyperglycaemia and osmotic diuresis and simultaneously to uncontrolled breakdown of fatty acids resulting in raised levels of ketone bodies (Williams & Pickup, 1992). Ketoacidosis is most frequently seen in newly diagnosed diabetics where it is often the presenting problem, in cases where insulin therapy is discontinued such as in patient non-compliance or in intercurrent illness.

The clinical features of ketoacidosis include:

■ polyuria, nocturia and polydipsia;
■ weight loss and feelings of weakness;
■ cramps – abdominal and leg;
■ nausea and vomiting;
■ visual disturbances;
■ drowsiness and confusion;
■ coma;
■ ketone breath (not always present/recognisable).

Ketoacidosis represents an urgent clinical problem and patients will require hospitalisation. Investigations include measurement of blood glucose, ketones and urea and electrolytes, including pH. Blood gases are required if the patient is in shock. Identification of possible infection should be undertaken by culturing blood and urine specimens (Drury, 1986; Williams & Pickup, 1992).

The clinical management of ketoacidosis involves:

■ rehydration, via intravenous infusion;
■ reduction and close monitoring of blood glucose;
■ correction of biochemical abnormalities;
■ treatment of intercurrent illness.

Prevention of ketoacidosis is extremely important and patients should be made aware of its seriousness. An extremely common cause of ketoacidosis is discontinuation of insulin therapy when the patient is not eating or is vomiting (Paterson, 1990). Patients need to be advised against this. Accidental underdose of insulin as a result of poor injection technique may give rise to ketoacidosis. Intentional withdrawal from insulin as an act of defiance in teenagers and young adults may also be a cause of ketoacidosis.

Foot problems

Some 5% of diabetics experience chronic foot problems associated with neuropathy, whilst 0.5% of patients will develop gangrene (World Health Organisation, 1985). A number of features of diabetes predispose the patient to foot problems. Elderly people, who may already have problems caring for their feet, are especially at risk (Paterson, 1990). Good foot care is essential and the involvement of community nurses and of chiropodists can be invaluable in this respect.

Care of diabetic patients' feet should aim primarily at prevention of problems. However, prompt and appropriate treatment, with the involvement of relevant specialists, chiropodists, neurologists and vascular surgeons, is vital. The common types of problems seen are corns, ulcers, ischaemia, sometimes with gangrene, and infections. These problems typically arise as a result of some form of trauma, which may be mechanical (ill-fitting shoes), chemical (corn remedies) or caused by heat (hot water bottles or heating pads).

Foot malformation is common in people with diabetes as a result of such factors as oedema, prior amputation and 'charcot joints' (a classic pattern of damage and disorganisation seen in diabetic feet). This can result in abnormal stresses on the foot and difficulty in getting shoes which fit well.

Patients should be taught to care for and regularly inspect their feet (Paterson, 1990). The following are points of special importance:

- Cut toenails straight across and carefully; if cutting toenails is a problem get assistance.
- Never cut corns, or apply over the counter corn remedies.
- Seek proper specialist attention for even apparently minor foot problems.
- Wear comfortable, well fitting shoes and seek specialist advice if it is difficult to get shoes which fit.
- Never go barefoot, even indoors.
- Wash feet daily and dry thoroughly, especially between the toes. Apply medicated talc and, if skin is dry, an appropriate emollient.

- Inspect feet daily for signs of calluses, blisters, breaks, discoloration or infection. (Prompt attention should be sought for any of these.)
- Avoid bed heating devices (e.g. hot water bottles and heating pads). Use bed socks.
- Hand test bath and wash water before immersion of the feet.

Foot inspection should form part of any diabetic clinic visit. Health care professionals should seek to prevent damage, prevent or promptly treat infection, maintain or improve blood supply and ensure good diabetic control (Drury, 1986). Where lesions do occur treatment involves debridement, cleansing, treatment of infection and re-distribution of pressure. This in extreme circumstances may need to be through application of a plaster cast or bed-rest (Paterson, 1990).

Surgery and medication

Surgery on diabetic patients can be accomplished without problems but requires careful planning. Patients are often admitted early in order to ensure good pre-operative blood glucose control, since the stress of surgery increases the risk of hyperglycaemia and ketoacidosis. In patients with NIDDM having minor surgery, monitoring alone may be sufficient. In IDDM patients or in major surgery on NIDDM patients an infusion of glucose, potassium and insulin is required, which will start before surgery and be carried on through and after surgery (Williams & Pickup, 1992). Blood glucose will need to be carefully monitored throughout.

Dentistry can be undertaken without any special preparation unless general anaesthetic is required, whereupon a referral to the dental hospital is suggested (Watkins, 1993). The increased risks of respiratory arrest in diabetic patients after drugs which suppress respiration, such as anaesthetics and opiates, need to be taken into account.

The effects of some drugs on oral hypoglycaemics have been discussed previously. Other important points about medication and diabetes which require consideration are:

- Always bear in mind potential drug interactions – check for these in the *British National Formulary* when a patient starts a new drug.
- Thiazine diuretics should not be given in

NIDDM, since they strongly promote hypergly-caemia (Williams & Pickup, 1992).

- Sugar-containing over the counter drugs are considered to be acceptable in the short, but not the long term (Caird, 1990).

Non-compliance with treatment

As with any long term health problem, treatment non-compliance is commonly seen in diabetes. Particular areas of diabetic care in which compliance problems are found include:

- Dietary non-compliance (Knight, 1990b). Reasons include poor understanding, anxieties about cost, and unwillingness to change behaviour.
- False recording by patients of blood and urine glucose values (Watkins, 1993).
- Defiance, especially in teenagers (Watkins, 1993); and attempts to manipulate health care professionals (e.g. to gain hospital admission).

Appropriate interventions from health care professionals may include assessment of self-management techniques and remedial education; alteration of regimen; and identification of anxiety or distress resulting in deviation from the prescription. It is important to note that punitive approaches may have the negative effect of forcing patients to conceal potentially life-threatening problems.

There is a significant correlation between good glycaemic control and reduction of complication rate. However, it is also important that diabetic complications should not automatically be ascribed to non-compliance since, as Walker (1993) points out, complications can be seen even in patients with very good glycaemic control.

Pregnancy

The risks involved for women who are diabetic and pregnant have declined in recent years, for both mother and baby. However, pregnancy in diabetes does still carry risks over and above those faced by the general population. Maternal mortality may be slightly higher than in the general population and women with diabetes are more likely to require Caesarean section (Williams & Pickup, 1992). Pregnancy may exacerbate existing diabetic problems like retinopathy and nephropathy (Drury, 1986). Control of blood sugar worsens in pregnancy. Hypoglycaemia is reported to be common in the early months of pregnancy.

There are a number of risks to the babies of diabetic mothers:

- In utero death and congenital malformation during ketoacidotic episodes.
- Increased risk of stillbirth.
- Increased incidence of neonatal jaundice and respiratory distress syndrome.
- Hypoglycaemia is also common.
- The babies of diabetic mothers are typically macrosomic, i.e. heavier and longer than average.
  (Drury, 1986; Williams & Pickup, 1992)

Care of the diabetic mother-to-be requires a good team approach. The importance of good glycaemic control needs to be emphasised and regular monitoring for hypertension and proteinuria (possibly as often as weekly) will be required. Frequent ultrasound monitoring of foetal growth is desirable (Watkins, 1993). The aim should be for the mother to go to full term and have a vaginal delivery unless there are clear indications otherwise.

Insulin and dextrose infusions are normally given during labour. Close post partum monitoring is required because of the increased likelihood of hypoglycaemia. Breast feeding is encouraged, but will require a higher carbohydrate and fluid intake.

Lifestyle considerations

Diabetes can affect a number of areas of the patient's lifestyle, although plainly the degree will depend upon the severity of the patient's illness. The British Diabetic Association is a good source of advice on lifestyle implications of diabetes and how to deal with them. Common areas affected are:

- Work
- Travel
- Hobbies
- Alcohol consumption
- Smoking
- Driving
- Insurance
- Family planning.

Work

Some patients are so severely debilitated that they are unable to work; others experience employment-related problems because of assumptions made by employers. Certain occupations are not open to diabetics (especially those with IDDM) because of the risk which would be entailed if they were to have a hypoglycaemic episode. These are typically occupations which include driving or flying. Shift work can have an adverse effect on glycaemic control.

Travel

Glycaemic control may be affected if the patient experiences such problems as sea sickness (for which the usual remedies may be used) or diarrhoea. The patient will need to ensure that adequate supplies (including emergency carbohydrate) and spare equipment (in case of loss or breakage) is taken. Refrigeration of insulin is only essential in very hot climates. Equipment should be kept in hand luggage; when travelling by plane insulin should never be stored in the hold as it may freeze. If travelling westward by plane, the patient may need to take additional short acting insulin followed by food (Williams & Pickup, 1992).

Hobbies

Exercise is actively encouraged in diabetics. IDDM patients need to be aware of the need to take precautions against hypo or hyperglycaemia when exercising. Williams and Pickup (1992) suggest taking an extra 20–40 g of carbohydrate before exercise and at hourly intervals during exercise. Alternatively, insulin can be reduced by between 30 and 50% before exercise. Close monitoring of blood glucose is required and patients should be aware that post-exercise hypoglycaemia can still occur the day after exercise. Patients with NIDDM do not usually need to increase carbohydrate intakes and post-exercise hypoglycaemia is reportedly uncommon in these patients. Patients need to be aware of the risk of hypoglycaemia when choosing hobbies and some dangerous sports may be inadvisable. Patients who are unsure whether a sport or hobby is suitable should seek professional advice.

Alcohol

Moderate alcohol intake is acceptable (except in patients with symptomatic neuropathy or high blood triglyceride levels), but should not be more than three units daily for men and two for women. Alcohol causes hypoglycaemia and may prolong the effects of sulphonylureas. Drinking before driving is to be avoided. High calorie alcoholic beverages (e.g. sweet wines or liqueurs), mixers and 'diabetic' beers are not recommended.

Smoking

Smoking is even more harmful for diabetics than for the general population and greatly increases the risk of cardiovascular disease, stroke and amputation. All diabetics should be strongly advised against smoking and the appropriate help given to those who wish to stop smoking.

Driving

Hypoglycaemia and visual impairment are the factors most likely to affect a diabetic patient's ability to drive or to hold a driving licence. All diabetic patients are required by law to notify the Driver and Vehicle Licensing Authority (DVLA) of their condition and will only be given a driving licence on receipt by the DVLA of a certificate of fitness from the GP. Similarly, the company giving vehicle insurance must be told (Drury, 1986). Patients need to check their blood glucose before a journey and to pull over at the first signs of a hypoglycaemic episode. It is essential that readily accessible emergency carbohydrate be carried.

Insurance

Insurers need to be told of the patient's condition and may increase premiums. It is worthwhile for the patient to contact the British Diabetic Association before seeking insurance, as it has lists of brokers who can obtain optimum rates for diabetics. Life insurance is a worthwhile investment for diabetics, owing to their below average life expectancy and can help to reduce financial hardship for families should premature death occur.

Family planning

Pregnancy was formerly not advised in women with diabetes. However, this is no longer generally the case, and only those with severe diabetic complications or very poor obstetric histories are advised against becoming pregnant. A pre-planned pregnancy, with good glycaemic control established before conception is preferred (Drury, 1986).

Most forms of contraception may be used by diabetic women with little increased risk above that of non-diabetic women, although the usual cardiovascular risk factors associated with oral contraceptive pills need to be borne in mind. High-dose oestrogen preparations should not be used (Williams & Pickup, 1986). If pregnancy is contraindicated, oral contraceptives are preferred over other methods as their failure rate is lower; sterilisation of either partner may also be considered. Impotence is common in men with diabetes. Many people with diabetes worry about the risk of passing the condition on to their children. Although there is some evidence that diabetes can be inherited (Martin & Knight, 1990) the likelihood appears to be low. Drury (1986) gives inheritance risks for IDDM of 2% if one parent has IDDM and 10% if both do so. People with diabetes should not be discouraged from having children on the sole grounds of inheritance risk for children.

Patient education in diabetic management

Patient education is considered to be crucial to successful self-management of diabetes and there is evidence of the positive impact of patient education in improving glycaemic control and reducing the incidence of such complications as foot problems (Knight, 1990b; Walker, 1993). The educative process is not a simple one (see Chapter 14).

The British Diabetic Association has produced guidelines for patient educators as to the minimum information necessary for safe patient self-management and the major topic areas are:

- Type of diabetes
- Therapy and its rationale
- Dietary guidance
- Hypo and hyperglycaemia
- Monitoring and control
- Complications
- Foot care
- Intercurrent illness

There are a number of teaching aids available, many from the British Diabetic Association, which can assist in formulating creative patient education strategies. In addition many hospitals now have specialist diabetic centres from which information can be obtained, and liaison with a diabetic specialist nurse is worthwhile before undertaking diabetic patient education.

Community nurses have an important role to play in the management of diabetic patients. Research evidence suggests that good diabetic management can have a significant impact in reducing morbidity and long term health problems for this patient group. Investment in good diabetic care therefore has clear potential to improve patient outcomes and also to provide manpower and cost benefits for the health service.

10.6 SUMMARY

Approximately 1–2% of the population have diabetes mellitus. There are two main types of diabetes, insulin dependent and non–insulin dependent. If diabetes is not well controlled then a number of long term complications may arise such as retinopathy, nephropathy or vascular problems. Much damage is preventable or reversible if detected early. The aims of diabetic management are threefold:

(1) symptom relief;
(2) hypoglycaemia and ketoacidosis prevention;
(3) prevention and delay or control of complications.

Management of diabetes is primarily concerned with keeping blood glucose values as close to physiological norms as possible. There is an association between good control and the prevention of diabetic complications. The principal means of controlling blood glucose are diet, oral hypoglycaemia and insulin. The level of diabetic control can be maintained by urine testing and monitoring of capillary blood glucose.

As with any long term health problem, treatment non-compliance is commonly seen. The community nurse is regularly involved in the administration of insulin to patients and in the assessment of self-management techniques. It is important to note that punitive techniques may have a negative effect of forcing patients to conceal potentially life-threatening symptoms. It is important that diabetic complications should not automatically be attributed to non-compliance.

Patient education is considered to be crucial to the successful self-management of diabetes and community nurses have a key role to play in this area.

10.7 REFERENCES AND FURTHER READING

American Diabetic Association (1993) *Report on the Diabetes Control and Complications Trial* American Diabetes Association, New York.

British Diabetic Association (1992) *Dietary Recommendations for People with Diabetes: an Update for the 1990's* British Diabetic Association, London.

Caird, F.I. (1990) General prescribing problems in elderly diabetic patients. In *Diabetes in Elderly People – A Guide for the Healthcare Team* (Ed. by C.M. Kesson & P.V. Knight) Chapman and Hall, London.

Drury, M.I. (1986) *Diabetes Mellitus* (2nd ed) Blackwell Scientific Publications, Oxford.

Helgason, T. & Jonasson, M. (1981) Evidence for a food additive as a cause of ketosis–prone diabetes, *Lancet*, **2**, 716–20.

Kelleher, D. (1988) *Diabetes* (part of the Experience of Illness series; series editors Fitzpatrick, R. & Newman, S.) Routledge, London.

Kesson, C.M. (1990) Shared care. In *Diabetes in Elderly People – A Guide for the Healthcare Team* (Ed. by C.M. Kesson & P.V. Knight) Chapman and Hall, London.

Knight, P.V. (1990a) Oral therapy. In *Diabetes in Elderly People – A Guide for the Healthcare Team* (Ed. by C.M. Kesson & P.V. Knight) Chapman and Hall, London.

Knight, P.V. (1990b) Education of elderly people with diabetes. In *Diabetes in Elderly People – A Guide for the Healthcare Team* (Ed. by C.M. Kesson and P.V. Knight) Chapman and Hall, London.

Knight, P.V & Kesson, C.M. (1990) Introduction – a short guide to some salient points. In *Diabetes in Elderly People – A Guide for the Healthcare Team* (Ed. by C.M. Kesson & P.V. Knight) Chapman and Hall, London.

Martin, B.J. (1990) Monitoring control of diabetes in the elderly patient. In *Diabetes in Elderly People – A Guide for the Healthcare Team* (Ed. by C.M. Kesson & P.V. Knight) Chapman and Hall, London.

Martin, B.J. & Knight, P.V. (1990a) Epidemiology and pathophysiology – who, where, what and why? In *Diabetes in Elderly People – A Guide for the Healthcare Team* (Ed. by C.M. Kesson & P.V. Knight) Chapman and Hall, London.

Martin, B.J. & Knight, P.V. (1990b) Clinical features and case detection – listening, looking and investigating. In *Diabetes in Elderly People – A Guide for the Healthcare Team* (Ed. by C.M. Kesson & P.V. Knight) Chapman and Hall, London.

National Kidney Research Fund (1987) *Diabetes Mellitus and Renal Disease* National Kidney Research Fund, London.

Paterson, K.R. (1990) Foot care. In *Diabetes in Elderly People – A Guide for the Healthcare Team* (Ed. by C.M. Kesson & P.V. Knight) Chapman and Hall, London.

Phillips, P.A. (1990) Dietary assessment and therapy. In *Diabetes in Elderly People – A Guide for the Healthcare Team* (Ed. by C.M. Kesson & P.V. Knight) Chapman and Hall, London.

Roberts, M. (1990) The role of the specialist nurse. In *Diabetes in Elderly People – A Guide for the Healthcare Team* (Ed. by C.M. Kesson & P.V. Knight) Chapman and Hall, London.

Walker, R (1993) Care and control of diabetes: finding the right balance, *Primary Health Care*, **3**, 10, 16, 18, 20.

Watkins, P.J. (1993) *The ABC of Diabetes* British Medical Association, London.

Williams, G. & Pickup, J.C. (ed.) (1992) *Handbook of Diabetes* Blackwell Scientific Publications, Oxford.

World Health Organisation (1985) *Diabetes Mellitus: Technical Report Series 727* WHO Publications, Geneva.

11

𝒪 Asthma

Anne-Louise Caress

Black (1992) describes asthma as being a syndrome rather than a disease, which affects the bronchi. Others define asthma as being a condition involving reversible airflow obstruction, or more fully

'a disease characterized by variable dyspnoea due to widespread narrowing of the airways in the lungs, varying in severity over short periods of time either spontaneously or as a result of treatment'

(Grant, 1982)

It is noted, however, that defining asthma is difficult, since the nature of the condition is not fully understood.

Prevalence of asthma

Prevalence estimates for asthma vary. Pearson (1993) suggests that up to 2 million adults (5% of the population) and 1 million children (10% of the population) may be affected by asthma. Charlton *et al.* (1991) give a higher figure of 6% of the adult population, whilst Hardy (1992) gives figures of between 1.8% and 6.7% of the adult population. Warner *et al.* (1989) state that 10% of children suffer from asthma. A prevalence study amongst 2503 children aged 7 and 11 years, based on parental report of symptoms, gave an overall prevalence of 9.5% (Clifford *et al.* 1989). The findings of this study confirmed other work in revealing a higher prevalence rate in boys than in girls at some ages.

Asthma is described by the Department of Health (1992) as being a cause of 'substantial ill health', with Pearson (1993) estimating that asthma results in 90 000 hospital admissions each year. Estimates of mortality show some agreement, the figure typically given being 2000 deaths per annum (Barnes, 1988; Charlton *et al.*, 1991; Pearson, 1993). Partridge (1991) suggests that this means one death occurs due to asthma every four hours, whilst Pearson (1993) notes that 50–60% of asthma deaths occur in those aged 60 or over.

Whilst estimates of the actual prevalence vary, there is agreement that asthma prevalence is increasing. The causes of this increase are uncertain (Hardy, 1992) and the following have been suggested as contributors:

- a change in the way in which asthma is classified in the International Classification of Diseases;
- greater recognition of asthma;
- environmental factors, for example, pollution by cars.

There is also agreement that there are too many deaths and too much disablement resulting from asthma. In part, this is considered to be the result of poor self-management by patients and undertreatment by health professionals (British Thoracic Society *et al.*, 1990a).

Aetiology of asthma

It is now widely recognised that the aetiology of asthma is multifactorial (Grant, 1982). In some individuals, it is possible to identify external (or extrinsic) factors which result in asthma, whilst in others, it is not possible to identify such factors clearly. Grant (1982) notes that all individuals in whom extrinsic factors can be identified as contributing to asthma will demonstrate antibody formation when exposed to common allergens. This compares with only 20% of the general population. The allergens most commonly associated with asthma are those which are inhaled, e.g. pollen, house dust mites, animal dander, feathers and fungi. Grant (1982) states that ingested allergens (e.g. milk, eggs, yeast or grain products) may be associated with asthma, but are less important than inhaled factors.

A number of other factors have been found to contribute to asthma (Black, 1992; Grant, 1982), namely:

- Drugs
- Tartrazine
- Dust
- Chemicals
- Respiratory infection
- Exercise.

Initially psychological factors were seen as the most important contributor to asthma. However, it is now recognised that asthma primarily results from physiological factors which can be exacerbated by stress and anxiety (Grant, 1982).

11.2 SYMPTOMS AND PRESENTATION OF ASTHMA

The bronchi of patients with asthma are hyperreactive as a result of inflammatory processes (British Thoracic Society et al., 1990a) and therefore increasingly likely to constrict. Inflammatory processes also result in oedema and mucus overproduction, which exacerbate the narrowing of the airways. The physical symptoms experienced by patients are therefore those which arise from bronchoconstriction:

- Shortness of breath
- Tightness in the chest
- Cough
- Wheeze

It is important to note that wheeze may be absent in patients with a very severe asthma attack, as the volume of air being expired may be too small to give rise to a wheeze (Black, 1992).

Owing to the distressing nature of the physical symptoms, patients may also experience mental anguish and anxiety (Black, 1992). This may include fear of dying as the result of an asthma attack.

Grant (1982) notes that the symptoms of asthma may be confused with those of some other respiratory conditions and with pulmonary oedema resulting from cardiac problems. Careful investigation is therefore required to confirm a diagnosis of asthma.

Asthma may be described as being chronic or acute. It is important to note that an acute episode may even be experienced by those with chronic symptoms. Furthermore, there is a small proportion of individuals who have so-called 'brittle' asthma (British Thoracic Society et al. 1990b). In these individuals, asthma becomes suddenly worse, with little or no advance warning for the patient (i.e. through deterioration in control). This is a very serious form of asthma, since an asthma attack can rapidly become life-threatening in these individuals. Warner et al. (1992) note that children with brittle asthma do not exhibit any abnormality in their lung function and show no symptoms other than during a bout of asthma.

Problems experienced by patients with asthma

Although asthma is usually a chronic condition, it is important to note that some patients will experience few episodes, whilst for others the condition will be severely debilitating. The range of problems experienced by patients therefore varies widely.

The main problem arising from asthma is shortness of breath and the limitations which this may impose. Areas of functioning which are commonly reported to be affected (Charlton et al. 1991) include:

- Mobility
- Exercise capability
- Work/school attendance
- Personal hygiene
- Social life

Shortage of circulating oxygen may result in exhaustion and dyspnoea on even minimal exertion. Severely affected patients may be limited to walking only a few yards before experiencing symptoms and climbing stairs may present difficulty. Early morning dyspnoea may hamper an individual's ability to wash and dress.

In some individuals, exercise itself may be the trigger for an asthma attack, known as exercise induced asthma (Black, 1992; Smith & Kendrick, 1993). Nonetheless, moderate exercise is noted as being important for asthmatic patients in helping to improve their control (Hardy 1992).

Charlton *et al.* (1991) collected data from a small sub-sample of 42 patients and found that more than 30% of these had lost time from school or work. Grant (1982) states that some individuals may become sensitised to allergens in their work environment, with resultant asthma. In these individuals, a change of work environment may be required.

Some patients may experience lifestyle limitations, notably in the area of socialising, especially in places like pubs and clubs where the atmosphere may be smoky. Social isolation is often experienced by patients with limited mobility. Partridge (1991) notes that some individuals with mild or infrequent episodes of asthma may nonetheless feel abnormal and be hampered by this.

11.3 GUIDANCE FOR PRACTICE – MANAGEMENT OF ASTHMA

There is a consensus that good management of asthma is vital in preventing unnecessary death and morbidity (British Thoracic Society *et al.*, 1990b; Charlton *et al.*, 1991; Rees, 1984; Warner *et al.*, 1992). It is also widely recognised that under-treatment is an important problem and results from both poor patient self-management and from failure by health care professionals to recognise and treat asthma adequately. Failure by patients to recognise the importance of worsening symptom control or by health care professionals to recognise the seriousness of an acute episode of asthma can be potentially fatal (British Thoracic Society *et al.*, 1990b).

Essential features of good asthma management are that the programme be structured and that patients receive good quality education. In addition effective and regular monitoring of lung function is desirable.

Management differs in acute and chronic asthma. For example, in chronic asthma, the aim is to use the lowest dose of medication possible to prevent symptoms (British Thoracic Society *et al.*, 1990a), whilst during a severe acute episode of asthma, high dose therapy is required (British Thoracic Society *et al.*, 1990b). Authoritative guidelines exist for the management both of adult and childhood asthma (British Thoracic Society *et el.*, 1990a and 1990b; Warner *et al.*, 1989 and 1992). All community nurses involved in the management of patients with asthma should familiarise themselves with these guidelines.

Aims of asthma management

The aims of asthma management are to:

- reduce morbidity and mortality;
- maintain normality in the patient's life;
- enable patients to manage their condition.

The two main planks of asthma management are patient education and pharmacological intervention.

Pharmacological management of asthma

The drugs used to manage asthma may be employed to reverse symptoms during an asthma episode and to prevent asthma symptoms (i.e. prophylactically). The extent to which a particular agent will serve in each of these functions depends upon its mode of action, duration of action and speed of action. All pharmacological agents used in the management of asthma are used to reduce bronchoconstriction in one or another way. In addition, patients may require antibiotics to treat chest infections, prompt treatment of infection being important in minimising exacerbation of asthma. The main groups of medications used are bronchodilators, non-steroidal prophylactic agents and corticosteroids (Black, 1992; British Thoracic Society *et al.*, 1990a).

Bronchodilators
The main groups of bronchodilators are:

- B$_2$-Agonists, e.g. salbutamol (Ventolin); terbutaline (Bricanyl); salmeterol (Serevent). These drugs act on the B-receptors responsible for causing smooth muscle relaxation (Smith & Kendrick, 1993).

■ Anticholinergics, e.g. ipratropium bromide (Atrovent). Anticholinergics inhibit the action of acetylcholine, which is a bronchoconstrictor.

■ Xanthines, e.g. theophyllines. Mode of action as bronchodilator unknown. Effect variable between individuals. Rate of metabolism affected by numerous factors (e.g. age, weight, other medications). Now considered to be useful only as second line therapy.

Non-steroidal prophylactics
■ Sodium chromoglycate stabilises the membranes of mast cells, thus preventing the triggering of an immune response.

■ Nedocromil has anti-inflammatory properties and inhibits the release of mediators of inflammation in the bronchial tract.

Corticosteroids
■ Corticosteroids (e.g. Prednisolone) have an anti-inflammatory effect. This results in diminution of bronchial hyper-reactivity; reduction in mucus secretion; and reversal of mucosal oedema.

Side effects and cautions

Anti-cholinergic agents have relatively few side effects (Smith & Kendrick, 1993). Those which are seen include retention of urine, exacerbation of glaucoma, dry mouth and blurring of vision.

Xanthines are reported to give rise to such problems as gastro-intestinal disturbance, headache and increased urine output. It is important to note that toxicity of this drug may be easily induced (Black, 1992) and can be potentially fatal.

No important side effects are noted for non-steroidal prophylactic agents. Coticosteroids, however, have numerous adverse effects (Black, 1992; Warner *et al.*, 1992) notably:

■ Growth retardation in children
■ Diabetogenesis
■ Skin problems
■ Fluid retention
■ Gastric ulceration
■ Muscle wasting and osteoporosis
■ Hypertension
■ Mood disturbance.

It is typically the case that the likelihood of adverse effects of asthma treatment will increase as the drug dose increases.

11.4 GUIDANCE FOR PRACTICE – ADMINISTRATION OF ASTHMA MEDICATIONS

The routes of administration of medications used in the treatment of asthma are:

■ Inhalation
■ Nebulisation
■ Oral administration
■ Intravenous administration.

It is considered preferable where possible to give inhaled medications. This route of administration enables delivery of drugs directly to their required site of action; consequently, medication doses may be reduced and side effects minimised (Barnes, 1988; British Thoracic society *et al.*, 1990a).

Most patients will use a metered dose administration device. However, problems with the use of these are noted (Warner *et al.*, 1992). For example, as many as 50% of children may exhibit poor inhaler technique. For younger patients or adults with poor co-ordination of drug administration and inhalation, alternatives include a spacer device or dry-powder inhalation system (e.g. Rotohaler). A spacer device may also be useful for emergency administration of medications during an acute asthma attack (e.g. 20–50 puffs of salbutamol) in the absence of a nebuliser (British Thoracic Society *et al.*, 1990b). Use of the spacer may enable continuation of low dose therapy and may reduce side effects if high dose therapy is required.

Inhaler technique

When using a standard metered dose device, proper technique is crucial to successful medication. It is important that patients perform the procedure described in Table 11.1.

Patients need to ensure that the inhaler device is kept clean and free from dust (hence the importance of re-capping); that the device is functioning properly; and, importantly (especially for those with episodic asthma who may only use inhalers infrequently) that the medication has not expired. The medication vial may be turned around or if necessary temporarily removed from the inhaler device in order to check

Table 11.1 Inhaler technique.

- Remove cap from inhaler.
- Expire fully.
- Place inhaler mouthpiece in mouth and press lips firmly around mouthpiece.
- Activate device and simultaneously inhale.
- Continue inhaling until lungs are fully inflated.
- Hold breath for a count of ten.
- Wait for a short period and then repeat the procedure.
- Recap the inhaler device.

this, but must be carefully replaced and a check made to ensure that the device still functions correctly.

Nebulisation

Nebulisation may be required for:

- the very young;
- those who are too dyspnoeic to inhale medications;
- those with poor inspiratory effort;
- those with poor co-ordination.

Important points in the administration of medications via a nebuliser include:

- ensuring an airflow of at least 6 litres/min;
- ensuring sufficient volume in chamber to allow for residual volume of 0.5 ml. Hughes (1989) recommends a minimum of 3 ml;
- appropriate cleaning and storage of the nebuliser;
- regular maintenance of equipment and observation for problems, for example overheating due to unusually long administration times (should be 7–10 minutes).

Dale (1987) reports the findings of a study which demonstrated bacterial contamination in nebuliser chambers which were rinsed with tap water and suggests therefore that tap water should not be used for this purpose unless boiled. It is further suggested that nebuliser equipment be stored dry.

Administration of nebulisers

Nebulisation involves the formation of a fine mist of particles (aerosol) containing medication. The mist is formed by agitation of a solution which has been placed within an appropriate delivery device, i.e. a nebuliser chamber. The source of the agitation is a stream of oxygen or air. Air may come from a cylinder or be provided by an air compressor. The patient uses a face mask or mouthpiece attached to the nebuliser chamber to allow the aerosol to be inhaled. The correct technique for nebuliser therapy is as follows:

Preparation of equipment
Attach the delivery tubing to the nozzle of the oxygen or air supply and check that the nebuliser chamber is attached to the delivery tubing. If an air compressor is being used, the device must be connected to a mains supply and the mains supply switched on.

Preparation of medication
Place the medication in the bowl of the nebuliser chamber. Solutions may come in separate ampoules pre-prepared with a single medication dose. Alternatively, the solution may be bottled concentrate, which will require dilution with saline or sterile (not tap) water. This will require that the patient have needles and syringes with which to draw up the solution. Tuition in the technique of drawing up solutions will be required.

Positioning of patient
Patients should get into a comfortable position, sitting upright or, if in bed, in as upright a position as possible. They should be well-supported with pillows as they will have to remain in this position until the end of the procedure. Small children may be best seated on an adult's lap.

Using the equipment

Place the mask over the nose and mouth. Switch on the compressor or open the valve to the air/oxygen supply. A fine mist should become visible.

Inhalation

Patients should breathe as deeply and evenly as possible throughout the therapy and keep the mask or mouthpiece *in situ*, removing it only to clear excess sputum in order to prevent blockage of equipment. Nebulisation should be complete in approximately 10 minutes.

After treatment has finished

The mask or mouthpiece should be wiped clean and all parts of the equipment appropriately stored. Hughes (1989) recommends daily cleansing of the nebuliser chamber (or after each treatment for viscous solutions); weekly cleansing of delivery tubing and weekly replacement of syringes and needles, with proper disposal of needles.

As with other inhaled medications, it is important that patients be taught to check expiry dates and to store agents correctly and safely.

Other routes

Oral therapy may be administered in tablet or linctus form. This is especially common as a route of administration for xanthines and steroids and is typically used for medications given to support inhaled therapy and for prophylaxis.

The other systemic route of drug administration is the intravenous route. This route is reserved for the treatment of severe, acute asthma (British Thoracic Society *et al.*, 1990b), and medications given intravenously include steroids and aminophylline.

11.5 OTHER ASPECTS OF ASTHMA MANAGEMENT

The importance of using objective measures to aid asthma diagnosis and management are stressed by the British Thoracic Society (1990). These include:

- Reversibility testing (i.e. resolution of symptoms after trial of anti-asthma medication).
- Peak expiratory flow measurement.
- Drug usage.
- In acute severe asthma, respiratory rate, heart rate and blood gases.

Peak flow measurement

Peak flow measurement is considered to be invaluable in the assessment of asthma control. Deteriorating peak flow readings are suggestive of worsening control, even in patients who do not subjectively perceive a deterioration in their condition. It is suggested that patients be advised to consider changes in peak flow in terms of the proportion of their usual best performance, rather using generalised reference values (British Thoracic Society *et al.*, 1990b). A peak flow reading which is 75% or less of the patient's usual best value is a cause for concern. (For the guidance of health professionals, this typically equates with a peak flow of less than 300 l/min.)

Peak flow measurement may also be used as a guide to the efficacy of therapy. It is invaluable in the management of an acute asthma episode. Regular recording of peak flow measurements before and after drug therapy will give a record of the medication's effectiveness. Furthermore, wide diurnal variation in peak flow measurements is suggestive of poor control or a deterioration in condition (Black, 1992).

11.6 SELF-MANAGEMENT OF ASTHMA

It is increasingly recognised that, where possible, patients (or their parents in the case of young children) should undertake most of the management of their condition, with health care professionals providing support (Barnes, 1988).

Community management of asthma has in fact become widespread, and many general practices run asthma clinics where newly diagnosed patients are educated and all patients regularly followed up. Warner *et al.* (1992) suggest that the management team should involve doctors, nurses and physiotherapists. Dietitians may also be involved in the care of debilitated, chronically ill patients. The importance of ensuring that patients with asthma are cared for by a doctor with some expertise in asthma management is stressed by the British Thoracic Society *et al.* (1990a).

The importance of community nursing involvement in the management of asthma is widely recognised (Barnes, 1988; Charlton *et al.*, 1991). As with other chronic conditions, it is important that nurses have relevant skills and training to care for patients with asthma (Barnes, 1988). The value of nurse-run asthma clinics was demonstrated by Charlton *et al.* (1991) in a study involving 115 asthmatic patients in a single general practice. The nurses had undergone a short period of relevant training and were involved in patient education and monitoring. It was found that patients experienced a reduction in their need for oral steroids, a fall in absences from school or work, and an overall reduction in morbidity, although the authors were unable to identify clearly which features of the clinic could account for these changes.

In a series of articles on nurse-run asthma clinics, Charlton (1989a and b) suggests the following as being important contributors to the success of the clinics:

- relevant nurse training;
- co-operation between nurse and doctor;
- provision of appropriate equipment (e.g. peak flow meters);
- clear identification of appropriate patients;
- good recording of each patient's asthma profile;
- formulation of individualised patient self-management plans according to clearly defined and agreed criteria.

Patient education

Patient education is the cornerstone of successful management of asthma (Barnes, 1988; British Thoracic Society *et al.*, 1990a; Partridge, 1991). Specific areas in which education is considered to be important include:

- Information about asthma including anatomy and physiology and trigger factors.
- Practical aspects including inhaler technique, peak flow monitoring and care of equipment (e.g. nebulisers).
- Differences between prevention and symptom relief. The importance of continuing to take

prophylactic therapies even when symptom free must be stressed.
- Recognition of decreasing control.
- Action to be taken in emergencies.
- Managing activities of daily living including advice on exercise, nutrition and stress-relieving techniques.

Self-management plans

The use of individualised self-management plans is increasingly commonplace and is considered to be an effective way of promoting better management of asthma (Charlton *et al.*, 1991; Partridge, 1991).

The goal of a self-management plan is to provide an individually tailored regimen which will result in the patient getting appropriate therapy in a variety of circumstances. The formulation of such a plan is contingent upon health care professionals having detailed and accurate advice about the patient's individual presentation of asthma. Grant (1982) suggests an asthma profile, which can be used to ensure that such data are obtained.

Self-management plans vary greatly in their complexity. A commonly used format is the asthma card provided by the National Asthma Campaign (British Thoracic Society *et al.*, 1990a; Partridge, 1991). These are available for both adults and children and for non-English speakers. Partridge (1991) notes that the complexity of a self-management plan will vary according to the capabilities of the patient; he suggests that a simple self-management plan would need to include the following:

- daily dose of prophylactic medication;
- name of the drug to be used if symptom breakthrough occurs;
- signs of deteriorating asthma control;
- advice on situations requiring an increase in therapy.

The British Thoracic Society *et al.* (1990a) suggest that a self-management plan should also include details on monitoring the condition. All patients should also be familiar with the action to be taken in case of emergency.

In the first instance the minimum advice given should be sufficient to enable the patient to recognise the difference between prevention and symptom relief. Secondly the patient should know how to recognise a deterioration in control and what action to take. Provision of explicit guidance is essential for patients with 'brittle' asthma, since their condition may rapidly become life-threatening.

11.7 ASTHMA CRISES

Any rapid deterioration in a patient's condition or failure to respond to therapy is serious and will require urgent medical attention and hospitalisation. The British Thoracic Society *et al.* (1990b) state that the presence of any of the following should be regarded as an emergency:

■ Respiratory rate of 25 breaths/minute or greater.
■ Heart rate persistently 110 beats/minute or greater.
■ Peak flow less than 40% of predicted normal or less than 200 l/min.
■ Fall in systolic blood pressure of 10 mmHg or more on inspiration.
■ A patient unable to complete a sentence in one breath or rise from lying/sitting due to increasing wheeze or dyspnoea.

If a patient shows signs of exhaustion, confusion or unconsciousness, is cyanosed or has a bradycardia then urgent treatment is necessary (British Thoracic Society, *et al.*, 1990a).

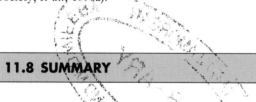

11.8 SUMMARY

Asthma has been identified as a source of high morbidity and mortality. The prevalence of the condition is increasing. Under-treatment results in substantial unnecessary suffering and requires attention from health care professionals to ensure that patients receive structured, appropriate management based on objective measurements. The role of patient education in successful asthma management is also stressed.

The contribution of community nurses in ensuring that patients receive such care is recognised. In order for their care of asthmatic patients to be fully effective, it is important that community nurses receive appropriate training and familiarise themselves with the relevant clinical guidelines.

11.9 REFERENCES AND FURTHER READING

Barnes, G. (1988) Asthma: latest developments in care, *Professional Nurse*, **4**, 364–8.

Black, P.A. (1992) Greater understanding enhances control, *Professional Nurse*, **8**, 1, 57–60.

British Thoracic Society, Research Unit of the Royal College of Physicians of London, King's Fund Centre and National Asthma Campaign (1990a) Guidelines for management of asthma in adults: I – chronic persistent asthma, *British Medical Journal*, **301**, 651–3.

British Thoracic Society, Research Unit of the Royal College of Physicians of London, King's Fund Centre and National Asthma Campaign (1990b) Guidelines for management of asthma in adults: II – acute severe asthma, *British Medical Journal*, **301**, 797–800.

Charlton, I., Charlton, G., Broomfield, J. & Mullee, M.A. (1991) Audit of the effect of a nurse-run asthma clinic on workload and patient morbidity in general practice, *British Journal of General Practice*, **41**, 227–31.

Charlton, I. (1989a) Setting up asthma clinics, *The Practitioner*, **233**, 1359–62.

Charlton, I. (1989b) Asthma clinics: how to run one, *The Practitioner*, **233**, 1440–45.

Clifford, R.D., Radford, M., Howell, J.B. & Holgate, S.T. (1989) Prevalence of respiratory symptoms among 7 and 11 year old schoolchildren and association with asthma, *Archives of Disease in Childhood*, **64**, 1118–25.

Dale, B.A.S. (1987) Bacterial contamination of home nebulisers (letter), *British Medical Journal*, **295**, 1486.

Department of Health (1992) *Health of the Nation: A Strategy for Health in England and Wales* (Cmnd, 1986) HMSO, London.

Grant, I.W.B. (1982) *Asthma* (6th ed.) Update Publications Ltd, London.

Hardy, S.G. (1992) Nursing implications of increasing asthma prevalence, *British Journal of Nursing*, **1**, 13, 653–9.

Hughes, B. (1989) Practical nebulisation, *Chemist and Pharmacy Update*, August 1989 bulletin.

Partridge, M.R. (1991) Self-care plans for asthmatics, *The Practitioner*, **235**, 715–21.

Pearson, M.G. (1993) Asthma guidelines: who is guiding whom and where to? *Thorax*, **48**, 3, 197–8.

Rees, J. (1984) *The ABC of Asthma* British Medical Association, London.

Smith, E.C. & Kendrick, A.H. (1993) How do inhaled bronchodilators work? *Professional Nurse*, 8, 8, 531–5.

Warner, J.O., Neijens, H.J. *et al.* (1992) Asthma: a follow-up statement from an International Paediatric Asthma Consensus Group, *Archives of Disease in Childhood*, 67, 240–48.

Warner, J.O., Gotz, M., Landau, L.I., Levison, H., Milner, A.D., Pedersen, S. & Silverman, M. (1989) Management of asthma: a consensus statement, *Archives of Disease in Childhood*, 64, 1065–79.

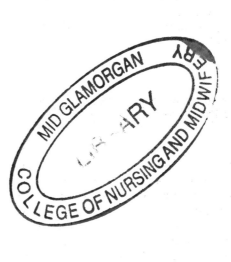

12

Screening Older People

Ann Pursey

12.1 INTRODUCTION

Universal assessment (screening) of older people for
their health and social care needs has been the subject
of much debate over the past 40 years. Recent discussions have been stimulated by the inclusion within
the 1990 general practitioner (GP) contract of a
statutory duty for GPs to offer an annual health check
and home visit to all patients aged over 75 years
registered with the practice (Health Departments of
Great Britain, 1989). Health visitors, district nurses
and practice nurses can all play key roles in the
assessment of health and social need in old age and
many are currently involved in screening or health
check programmes for people aged 75 and over.

12.2 BACKGROUND – THE AGEING POPULATION

Demographic changes

For the purposes of this chapter the 'onset of old age'
has as its starting point the chronological age of 65
years and over. Whilst not a very reliable predictor of
health status, it is currently the most widely used
definition.

Throughout the twentieth century the proportion
of people aged 65 and over has increased in all
countries of the world. In Great Britain, life expectancy this century has risen by more than 20 years

(Office of Population Censuses and Surveys, 1993).
The major causes of this rise are a reduction in child
mortality, particularly due to the prevention of
infectious diseases, and improvements in physical and
social environments. Improved medical treatment of
diseases once they have occurred and high-
technology interventions in health have had an impact
on life expectancy, albeit a limited one (Coleman *et al.*,
1993).

In population terms, there has been a gradual
decline in the number of people aged 65–74 years
relative to those aged 75 years and over. In 1981, 7%
of the total population was aged over 75 years whilst
the 65–74 age-group comprised 15.1% of the total.
The predicted percentages for 2001 are that 8.9% of
the population will be 75 years or over compared to
15.2% aged 65–74 years (Office of Population Censuses and Surveys, 1984, 1993). Proportionally,
therefore, the biggest increase in population terms
will be in the over 75 age group.

Within both age-groups there are more women
than men. The gender (sex) ratio at 85 years and over
is more than double that for the 65–74 age-group.
Owing to greater longevity and the tendency for
women to marry men older than themselves, women
are more likely to experience widowhood, to live alone
and to live in institutional settings (Arber & Ginn,
1991). Over the next 20 years there will also be a rapid
increase in the ageing of minority ethnic populations,
as those who migrated in the middle of this century
reach old age (Blakemore & Boneham, 1993).

Social changes

Approximately 95% of people aged 65 and over live in
the community (i.e. not in institutional settings) and it

has been estimated that, for every severely incapacitated older person living in an institution, there are four living in private households (Bond & Carstairs, 1982). Recent government policies have relied heavily on the notion of family care supporting older people at home in the community (Department of Health and Social Security, 1982; Secretaries of State for Health *et al.*, 1989). However, nearly one in three people aged 75 and over have no surviving children and the impact of divorce, geographical mobility, declining birthrate and the increase in the number of women in the workforce will all affect the availability of the family to care for ageing relatives. These trends will have important implications for the concept of community care.

Undoubtedly some older people require high levels of care from both relatives and the statutory services. However, it is important to recognise that older people themselves are frequently carers for other people. One research study found that the average age of the carers of confused old people was 61 years and that 30% of them were over 70 years (Levin *et al.*, 1988). There is a predicted increase in the trend for 'young old' people to be caring for 'old old' people.

The issue of the health and social needs of ethnic elders has only recently been discussed within research and policy literature and we currently know very little about ethnicity and its effect on health. Recent studies have demonstrated that, for example, Jewish older people express more functional difficulties than white Caucasian older people (Bowling *et al.*, 1991) and that the incidence of tuberculosis is higher in older people from Asian origins than in the Caucasian population. However, many of the problems experienced by people from other countries are to do with problems of lifestyle, e.g. difficulties in communicating in English (Donaldson & Odell, 1986), and lack of knowledge of available services and how to access them (Donaldson & Jackson, 1993).

12.3 HEALTH PROBLEMS AND AGEING

Many people associate old age with a time of ill-health. Research evidence shows that the majority of

people aged 65 years or more are not functionally impaired and that they live very independent lives in the community. In one study of 1406 people aged 65 and over, 93% believed their health to be fair to good for their age (Luker & Perkins, 1987). However, there is strong statistical evidence that with increasing age comes an increasing likelihood of functional and psychological impairment with three in five people aged over 85 years suffering a limiting long-standing illness.

Many of the functional problems that older people experience are relatively minor, yet they can have a significant effect on quality of life, and many of them are easily treatable. Yet older people frequently believe that they have functional problems because of their age and consequently do not seek medical or nursing advice and help. Screening has an important part to play in helping people to recognise that their health and social problems are frequently not a part of the 'normal ageing process' and that solutions and treatments for these problems can often be found.

The diversity of health problems experienced by older people warrants more in-depth description than is feasible in this chapter. Some of the common health problems faced by older people are briefly described here with key references given to guide the reader to more detailed discussions.

Hearing

Approximately one in three people aged 65 or over will have a hearing impairment. By the age of 75 years, this has risen to two in five people and by the age of 85 years approximately three in five people will have a hearing impairment (Office of Population Censuses and Surveys, 1984).

The first thing to establish when older people complain of deafness is whether their ears are clear of wax. The diagnosis of presbyacusis (the gradual deterioration in hearing ability associated with old age) is generally made by audiogram and if hearing loss is significant a hearing aid may be helpful. Hearing aids can be difficult to use effectively and people need adequate training and encouragement. Nurses can have an important role to play in training and educating older people to use their hearing aids correctly. Although deafness in old age is common it is often neglected and may be associated with psychiatric illness such as depression.

Vision

Presbyopia (where vision for distant objects is usually intact but close vision becomes blurred) is a feature of ageing experienced by the majority of the population over 65 years.

Over 90% of people aged 65 years and over wear glasses. However, 18–45% of them still have difficulty with vision in spite of wearing glasses. The percentage having difficulty increases with advancing age.

Nutritional status

There is an age component to nutritional status, although malnutrition is generally associated with significant mental impairment, physical illness or disability rather than with age *per se*. In general, absorption of food from the intestine is not significantly compromised by the ageing process. Most old people have an adequate intake of food although vitamin and trace element intake is often inadequate (Panel on Nutrition of the Elderly, 1972).

Some of the problems with eating and drinking arise from poor dental health. Many people aged 65 and over wear dentures and when these are ill-fitting they can severely impair an older person's ability to eat adequate amounts of food.

Pernicious anaemia is also a potential problem (due to decreased absorption of vitamin B12) for some individuals but this is easily solved by regular vitamin B12 injections. Constipation also presents a problem for some people and this is usually due to a general reduction in mobility and activity. Again, this is often easily solved by encouraging individuals to increase their intake of roughage.

Respiratory disease

Older people are more prone to respiratory infection and respiratory problems. There is a physiological deterioration in older lungs due to the normal ageing process and bronchitis is a commonly experienced health problem aggravated by poor housing conditions and problems with adequate heating. The incidence of asthma in the population as a whole is increasing and it is estimated that up to 90% of people aged 65 and over with asthma are undiagnosed. Chronic obstruction pulmonary disease (COPD) is also a feature of old age, particularly amongst smokers or ex-smokers. Severe chronic respiratory disease can have a devastating impact on lifestyle and activities.

Bones, muscles and mobility

Osteoporosis

Problems with bone density and thickness are marked in post-menopausal women. Osteoporosis affects many post-menopausal women making fractures more likely during a traumatic episode such as a fall. Continued physical activity and calcium supplements may help to minimise the onset or delay the progress of osteoporosis but treatment is not generally satisfactory.

Arthritis

Arthritis affects many people, the most common form being osteoarthritis which is mainly due to wear-and-tear of the large weight-bearing joints. Rheumatoid arthritis is a debilitating disease mainly affecting the small joints and treatment is mostly palliative (minimising the symptoms of pain and stiffness) although anecdotally there is thought to be a benefit from some forms of homeopathic treatment. In addition, there is emerging evidence that food allergies and constipation may have an impact on rheumatoid arthritis (both incidence and severity of disease).

Mental health and ageing

Cognitive decline

Cognitive decline is not usually marked before the age of 70 and is primarily determined by the processes of chronic physical disease, for example diabetes (Holland & Rabbitt, 1991). It is important to distinguish abnormal from normal psychological ageing. Memory deterioration (recent events particularly) may be marked in dementia, but there is little or no memory deterioration in the normal ageing process. Simple measures of learning show little or no decline into old age (Savage *et al.*, 1973). Mental function in old age must be considered in the context of an older person's life. Social isolation, sensory deprivation and lack of control over decision-making and the environment may all have a profound (but often reversible) effect on mental health. Psychological change with age is a complex issue to assess and requires an interdisciplinary approach which incorporates observation of the individual's behaviour.

Depressive illness

Depressive illness is the commonest mental health problem of old age. There is disagreement regarding the causes of depression in the older population. Certainly the degree of loss experienced by older people due to bereavement and changing life-events (such as retirement) should not be underestimated but there may also be a biological component to the incidence of depression in older people.

Dementia

Approximately one in fifty people aged 65 and over and one in five people aged 85 and over will have dementia. The majority of cases of senile dementia are due to Alzheimer's disease (a degenerative condition). The underlying cause of Alzheimer's disease has not been established to date although research is on-going. Another form of dementia is atherosclerotic dementia which is due to a series of small strokes. This accounts for about one in five people suffering dementia. The clinical diagnosis of these two conditions is often difficult, although in Alzheimer's dementia the deterioration in mental status tends to be more gradual than the series of step-like deteriorations in atherosclerotic dementia. The prevalence of depression and dementia among older people justifies the inclusion of questions about mental state in any assessment.

Medication

Older people often take a wide range of medicines, including non-prescription medicines (Anderson & Cartwright, 1986). In their review of medicines being taken by older people, Anderson and Cartwright (1986) found that GPs and the patients themselves tended to lack knowledge about the medicines prescribed. It is important that range and frequency of medicine used are established as the side-effects of particular drugs can have deleterious effects on older people.

Contact with health services

Ninety per cent of people aged over 75 consult their GP at least annually (Rogers, 1991) but this does not necessarily mean that their needs are being met. Many treatable conditions such as incontinence problems, difficulties with eyesight, hearing, teeth, feet, mobility and depression may not be reported by older people to their doctors.

Caring and older people

The needs of carers are well recognised in research literature, however it appears that caring for the carers is still not fully incorporated into health and social service provision. Given that a high number of older people are themselves caring for someone else, the consequences of care for and care by older people should be considered. When an assessment is conducted on an older person, the carer is generally only assessed on their ability to cope with the demands of caring and is therefore seen as of secondary importance to the primary focus of the assessment (the older person). Caring can have serious detrimental effects on people's health and therefore assessment of the carer's health needs should be an integral part of any in-depth assessment process.

Unmet need

There is evidence that under-reporting of ill-health and social need by older people still exists but recent research shows that this is a much smaller problem than was predicted ten years ago (Perkins, 1991). Farquhar & Bowling (1992) reviewed 23 published screening studies of people aged 65 and over by GPs and showed that in 20 of them 'unmet need' was indicated. Farquhar and Bowling showed that many people over 65 years were suffering from health problems which they had not consulted their GPs about. Eighty-five per cent of people had seen their GPs in the previous 12 months. The 15% of people who had not, tended to be amongst the healthiest of that population.

12.4 GUIDANCE FOR PRACTICE – SCREENING OLDER PEOPLE: APPROACHES AND TECHNIQUES

What is screening?

Screening has been defined by epidemiologists as the detection of pre-symptomatic abnormalities in a population (Department of Health and Social Security, 1977). By comparison, case finding is concerned with the early detection of symptomatic problems before they would normally be presented (Williamson, 1981; Taylor *et al.*, 1983).

Fig. 12.1 shows the range of approaches to case finding and screening. The emphasis within current screening programmes has moved from disease-detection to assessment of functional loss and consequently the role of the community nurse in functional assessments has increased in importance (Luker, 1982; Luker & Pursey, 1991).

Whilst general practitioners have been charged with the responsibility of offering these home visits, very frequently it is nurses (practice nurses, district nurses) or health visitors who carry out these assessments. In some areas unqualified link workers (who have received specific training) are undertaking the first stage health check (Wallace, 1990). It is important that whoever undertakes the assessment is adequately trained to do so (United Kingdom Central Council for Nursing, Midwifery and Health Visiting, 1990).

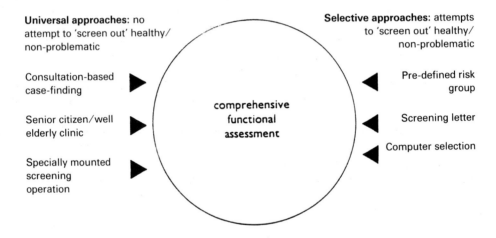

Figure 12.1 Screening and universal assessment. Source: Taylor R.C. & Buckley, E.G. (Eds) (1987) *Preventive Care of the Elderly: A Review of Current Developments.* Occasional Paper 35. London, Royal College of General Practitioners. Reproduced with permission of the publisher.

The 1990 General Practitioner Contract (Health Departments of Great Britain, 1989) outlines eight key assessment areas for universal screening of people aged 75 and over which are:

■ To see the home environment and to find out whether carers and relatives are available;
■ Social assessment (lifestyle, relationships);
■ Mobility assessment (walking, sitting, use of aids);
■ Mental assessment;
■ Assessment of the senses (hearing and vision);
■ Assessment of continence;
■ General functional assessment;
■ Review of medication.

(after the Health Departments of Great Britain, 1989)

A three-stage approach to screening

A three-stage approach to assessment is recommended as best practice:

(1) An initial health check screen;
(2) A fuller assessment of identified problems;
(3) A full interdisciplinary assessment.

(Williams & Wallace, 1993)

It is primarily during the first two stages that nurses working in the community are likely to be involved. The third stage assessment is likely to be interdisciplinary and would generally involve professionals from social services in addition to health care professionals. Whilst this may seem a lengthy process, there should, in fact, be relatively few individuals who require a full interdisciplinary assessment (Department of Health, 1992).

The benefit of a staged approach to screening and assessment is that the first stage can be used to screen out people who do not require a detailed assessment of health and social need. Research evidence for the number of people requiring follow-up varies from study to study. For example, Barber (1984) claimed that 80% of people aged 65 and over who completed a postal screening questionnaire in the first stage required a follow-up visit for further assessment. By comparison, Freer (1987) used the same screening schedule to guide consultations with older people and found that only 29% required a more in-depth assessment of health need. Nevertheless, a staged approach to assessment is recommended by most authors and researchers because it is more cost-effective than a universal in-depth assessment programme (Barber, 1984; Freer, 1987; Farquhar & Bowling, 1991; Luker & Pursey, 1991; Williams & Wallace, 1993).

Whilst the guidelines below pertain specifically to assessment of people aged 75 and over, they are entirely appropriate for professionals undertaking a screening programme with the 65–74 age-group.

Initial health check screen

The majority of GP practices have an age–sex register which enables the identification of clients within particular age-groups. The object of the initial screen is to identify those individuals with particular problems who will require a more in-depth assessment of their needs. The aim is therefore to identify the necessity for a more in-depth assessment, not necessarily to meet any needs identified.

Individuals may be contacted by letter, telephone or opportunistically (i.e. when an individual visits the practice/health centre or when a home visit is indicated for another reason). 'Cold-calling' (i.e. turning up at the house without making an appointment) is not recommended as it does not give the individual time to prepare for the visit and increases the risk of a high level of 'no access' visits. Poor response rates to letters inviting people to have a health check are generally due to the way the invitation is made (Williams & Wallace, 1993). The most important thing is that adequate explanation is given to the individual about the purpose and content of the assessment.

Health checks can be usefully performed in the practice or health centre or at the person's home. There are advantages to both settings and a flexible approach is recommended where individuals are given the choice of an assessment in the clinic or a home visit for assessment. The GP contract requires that a home visit is offered.

The GP contract provides an outline structure to guide assessments. However, interpretation of the assessment guidelines by different GP practices and primary health care teams is diverse. The checklists issued by some of the major drug companies are frequently used, though the degree to which the questions are based on research evidence of the needs of older people should be considered. The Royal College of General Practitioners' health check questionnaire is comprehensive yet simple and gives clear indication to the interviewer when a more in-depth assessment is needed (Williams & Wallace, 1993). It includes a brief financial assessment and a record of the services that an individual currently receives (see Section 12.8).

The issues that should be considered in an initial health check screen are as follows:

(1) Background information
- Age/date of birth
- Sex
- Last time the person was seen by a member of the practice
- Known clinical or social problems

(2) Home-environment and social circumstances
- Heating and warmth of the house
- Safety (in particular proneness to falls at home)
- Whether the person lives alone or with other people
- Whether the person is a carer or is cared for by someone
- Social contact with relatives and neighbours

(3) Mobility
- Ability to move around the house including up stairs/steps
- Ability to move around outside the house/to the shops, etc.

(4) General function
- Ability to do own shopping
- Ability to do housework and basic household repairs (e.g. changing a light-bulb)

- Ability to dress and undress themselves
- Ability to bath/shower or strip wash unaided

(5) Continence
Problems with urinary and faecal incontinence should be established. Attention needs to be given to stress incontinence and the link between mobility and problems getting to the toilet in time. (See also Chapter 8.)

(6) Hearing and vision
- Establish whether the person wears glasses and whether the person can see adequately, both long and short distances.
- Ability to hear, with or without a hearing aid.

(7) Mental function
The RCGP (Royal College of General Practitioners) recommend that the first stage assessment of psychological health combines a simple depression screening questionnaire (Shelk & Yesavage, 1986) and the Abbreviated Mental Test Score (AMTS) for dementia (Hodgkinson, 1972). (See Section 12.8.)

(8) Medication
- Find out which medicines people are taking and how often.
- Establish whether the person understands the reasons for taking each medicine.
- Establish what non-prescription medication the person also uses.

(9) Finances
- Establish whether the person has any problems paying their bills and has enough money for food.
- Sorting out finances.

(10) Receipt of services
- Establish what statutory/professional/voluntary services the person receives and the frequency of contact.

Opportunities arising from assessment and screening visits

Although the main aim of most screening programmes is to detect unmet health and social need in a population, the assessment visit provides opportunities for other issues concerning old people to be discussed. For well older people (or those whose health is under active supervision) the health check assessment can provide:

- reassurance that everything is alright;
- confirmation that health care professionals take an interest in older people;
- information about services that may be needed in the future and increased awareness of the support systems available (McEwan et al., 1990);
- further information about the GP practice and its facilities;
- the opportunity for primary prevention/health education advice
  (adapted from Williams and Wallace, 1993).

Research evidence shows that older people like and enjoy the assessment home visits and it is suggested that they may provide a boost in morale for older people who are not normally in contact with statutory services (McEwan et al., 1990). In addition, the visit offers the opportunity to discuss issues such as breast screening, cervical cytology, immunization, smoking, exercise, alcohol intake, accident prevention, etc., all of which are of potential importance and interest to older people.

An alternative to first home/clinic assessments

A viable alternative to face-to-face individual assessment is to write to individuals including a self-assessment to be returned to the practice or health centre.

There is clear research evidence that older people are capable of and willing to complete self-assessment questionnaires and that the response rate is generally high. In an average practice approximately 85–95% of people aged 75 and over who are sent a self-assessment questionnaire will return it (Bowns et al., 1991; Dowrick, 1993). One of the problems with self-assessments is the possibility that the non–responders are a high-risk group, i.e. people with high levels of unmet need (Bowns et al., 1991). However, this problem can be overcome by members of the primary health care team undertaking domiciliary visits by appointment to those who do not return the questionnaire.

Research studies have shown that self-assessment tools:

- are well validated (Barber, 1984; Pathy et al., 1992; Bowns et al., 1991).

- have been shown to have high sensitivity and specificity for predicting need and dependency when compared with structured interviews by research practice nurses (Bowns *et al.*, 1991).
- enable the identification of the need for services and unmet medical/health problems.
- provide a rapid means of screening out patients with no immediate health or social need.
- are a financially viable option as most GP practices already send out a letter of invitation for the current health check (Luker & Pursey, 1991).

Benefits of screening/health checks

For the past 20 years there has been considerable controversy about the benefits of screening and universal assessment programmes. It is interesting to note that elderly screening is now the focus of a large Medical Research Council randomised controlled trial. In a sense the debate is pointless whilst there is a statutory requirement within the GP contract for screening to be undertaken. The main benefit of a home visit is that the interaction with a health care professional appears to improve adaptation to old age and awareness of the support systems available (McEwan *et al.*, 1990). However there is little or no evidence of a resolution of physical problems or of improved ease with activities of daily living for older people who have been visited at home for assessment (McEwan *et al.*, 1990). There is evidence that screening is associated with a reduction in the amount of time spent in institutional care (Pathy *et al.*, 1992) although this is an area which requires further investigation.

Potential dangers of screening

Screening is not without its risks and nurses should consider the following issues carefully when planning or undertaking a screening programme with older people:

(1) There is a risk of highlighting problems that were not previously realised by the older people thereby raising their expectations that solutions to those problems will be found.
(2) The risk of intrusion of privacy is important and can be overcome by avoiding 'cold-calling' on people at home and by giving adequate explanation of the content and purpose of the assessments.

Record-keeping

Summaries of assessments should ideally be kept with the client's medical notes in the GP practice. Records should contain details of decisions made following the assessment, of referrals made and of action taken by the professional involved in undertaking the assessment. One of the problems with the check lists currently being issued by drugs companies is that they do not allow a comprehensive record of the assessment to be kept as much of the information is in the form of tick-boxes. Many people have developed a grid or table system on which problems identified in successive years can be quickly seen and progress or deterioration in each area can be monitored. The Royal College of General Practitioners' document *Health checks for people aged 75 and over* (Williams & Wallace, 1993) provides an example of a summary sheet that could be adapted to suit the needs of individual practices and practitioners. (See Section 12.8.)

Second and third stage assessments

When problems are identified following the first stage health check or self-assessment questionnaire, there is clearly a need for a more detailed assessment. In some cases, a full interdisciplinary assessment may be required at the earliest opportunity. At other times a more detailed assessment of a specific area of health need may be appropriate and may be performed by one professional (e.g. a community nurse) without reference to any other disciplines. Liaison with other agencies involved with the older person is vital at this stage, in order that essential information can be shared and exchanged.

It is not the intention of this chapter to describe the content of a second-stage assessment (see Williams & Wallace (1993) for an example of this). One area which is often neglected in assessments is the role of the carer in supporting the cared-for person at home.

It is important to remember that the older person being assessed may in fact be a carer too. In this context it is important to establish the basis of the relationship between carer and cared for person. Four key areas for assessment of the carer's needs include:

(1) Health
(2) Personal issues (related to their role as carer)

(3) Finances
(4) Household.

12.5 AUDIT AND QUALITY ISSUES

Clearly the efficacy of any screening programme will depend on:

- how accurately it identifies areas of need;
- the extent of coverage of the population. (Are those not screened the most in need?);
- consistency of approach of those involved in screening;
- acceptability to the target population.

It is possible to audit health checks on the following criteria:

- uptake of home visits/clinic visits;
- percentage return of self-assessment questionnaires;
- referrals made to other agencies/number of inappropriate referrals;
- time lag between referral and agency action;
- number of patients satisfied with the outcome of assessment/health check (this can be audited at each subsequent yearly visit);
- number of complaints received;
- number of second-stage assessments required.

There are many other, more specific, aspects of the health check, screening, and assessment system that could be audited. Perhaps the most important aspects to audit are whether the clients themselves were satisfied with the health check and whether any referrals made had the desired outcome.

12.6 SUMMARY

Many of the functional problems which older people experience are of a relatively minor nature, but they may have a significant influence on quality of life.

There has been a shift in emphasis in screening away from disease detection towards functional loss, and consequently the role of the community nurse in functional assessments has increased in importance.

The 1990 General Practitioner Contract (Health Departments of Great Britain, 1989) has given a prominence to health assessment for people of 75 years and over.

Whilst general practitioners have been charged with the responsibility of offering a home visit, very frequently it is nurses who carry out the assessment.

A three-stage assessment process is recommended as best practice:

(1) An initial health check screen;
(2) A fuller assessment of identified problems
(3) A full interdisciplinary assessment (Williams & Wallace, 1993).

It is in the first two stages that community nurses are likely to be involved. Whilst the GP contract provides an outline structure to guide assessments, interpretation of the assessment guidelines is variable. The Royal College of General Practitioners' health check questionnaire is comprehensive yet simple and gives clear indications to the interviewer when a more in-depth assessment is indicated (Williams & Wallace, 1993).

For over twenty years there has been considerable controversy about the benefits of screening and universal assessment programmes. There is evidence that screening is associated with a reduction in the amount of time spent in institutional care, although this is an area which requires further investigation.

12.7 REFERENCES AND FURTHER READING

Anderson R. & Cartwright A. (1986) The use of medicine by older people, In *Self-care and Health in Old Age. Health Behaviour. Implictions for Policy and Practice* (Ed. by K. Dean, T. Hickey & B.E. Holstein) Croom Helm, London.

Arber, S. & Ginn, J. (1991) *Gender and Later Life*. Sage Publications, London.

Barber, J.H. (1984) Screening and surveillance of the elderly at risk, *Practitioner*, **228**, 1389, 269–73.

Blakemore, K. & Boneham, M. (1993) *Age, Race and Ethnicity in Britain*. Oxford University Press, Milton Keynes.

Bond, J. & Carstairs V. (1982) *Services for the elderly: a survey of the characteristics and needs of a population of 5,000 old people*. Scottish Health Service Studies No. 42. Scottish Home and Health Department, Edinburgh.

Bowling, A., Farquhar, M. & Leaver, I. (1991) Ethnicity and ageing. Unpublished Working Paper.

Bowns, I., Challis, D. & Tong, M.S. (1991) Case finding in elderly people: validation of a postal questionnaire, *British Journal of General Practice*, 41, 344, 100–104.

Coleman, P., Bond, J. and Peace, S. (1993) Ageing in the twentieth century. In *Ageing in Society* 2nd edition (Ed. by J. Bond, P. Coleman & S. Peace) Sage Publications, London.

Department of Health and Social Security (1977) *Prevention and Health* (Cmnd 7047) HMSO, London.

Department of Health and Social Security (1982) *Ageing in the United Kingdom*. HMSO, London.

Donaldson, I.J. & Odell, A. (1986) Health and social status of elderly Asians: a community survey *British Medical Journal*, 293, 1079–82.

Donaldson, L. & Jackson, M. (1993) The health of older Asians, In *Ageing and Later Life*. (Ed. by J. Johnson & R. Slater) Sage Publications, London.

Dowrick, C. (1993) Self assessment by elderly people – a means of identifying unmet need in primary care, *Health and Social Care*, 1289–96.

Freer, C. (1987) Consultation-based screening of the elderly in general practice, *Journal of the Royal College of General Practitioners*, 37, 303, 455–6.

Farquhar, M. & Bowling, A. (1992) Older people and their GPs, *Journal of the British Society of Gerontology*, 2, 2, 7–10.

Health Departments of Great Britain (1989) *General practice in the National Health Service – the 1990 Contract* HMSO, London.

Hodgkinson, H.M. (1972) Evaluation of a mental test score for assessment of mental impairment in the elderly, *Age and Ageing*, 1, 233–8.

Holland, C.A. & Rabbit, P. (1991) The course and causes of cognitive change with advancing age, *Reviews in Clinical Gerontology*, 1 79–94.

Levin, E., Sinclair, I. & Gorbach, P. (1988) *Families, Services and Confusion in Old Age*. Gower, Aldershot.

Luker, K.A. (1982) *Evaluating Health Visiting Practice* Royal College of Nursing, London.

Luker, K.A. & Perkins, E.S. (1987) The elderly at home: service needs and provision, *British Journal of General Practice*, 37, 248–50.

Luker, K.A. & Pursey, A.C. (1991) *The nurse's role in assessment of the over 75s in general practice*. Geriatric Medicine Monograph, London.

McEwan, R.T., Davison, N., Forster, D.P., Pearson, P. & Stirling, E. (1990) Screening elderly people in primary care: a randomized controlled trial, *British Journal of General Practice*, 4094–7.

Office of Population Censuses and Surveys (1984) *Census Guide No. 1*. HMSO, London.

Office of Population Censuses and Surveys (1993) *Population Trends No. 71*. HMSO, London.

Panel on Nutrition of the Elderly (1972) *A Nutrition Survey of the Elderly*. DHSS Reports on Health and Social Subjects No. 3, HMSO, London.

Pathy, J., Bayer, A., Harding, K. & Dibble, A. (1992) Randomised trial of case finding and surveillance of elderly people at home, *The Lancet*, 340, 890–93.

Perkins, E.R. (1991) Screening elderly people: a review of the literature in the light of the new general practitioner contract, *British Journal of General Practice*, 41, 382–5.

Rogers, M. (1991) Screening elderly people. In *Towards Healthy Ageing: some nursing perspectives*. (Ed. by G. Garrett) Austen and Cornish, London.

Savage, R.D., Britton, P.G., Bolton, N. & Hall, E.H. (1973) *Intellectual Functioning in the Aged*. Methuen, London.

Secretaries of State for Health, Social Security, Wales & Scotland (1989) *Caring for People: Community Care in the Next Decade and Beyond* CM 849 (White Paper). HMSO, London.

Shelk, J.I. & Yesavage, J.A. (1986) Geriatric Depression Scale (GDS): recent evidence and development of a shorter version. In *Clinical Gerontology: A Guide to Assessment and Intervention* (Ed. by T.L. Brink) Howarth Press, New York.

Taylor, R., Ford, G. & Barber, H. (1983) *The Elderly at Risk*. Age Concern, London.

Taylor, R.C. & Buckley, E.G. (1987) *Preventive Care of the Elderly: a Review of Current Developments*. Occasional Paper 35. Royal College of General Practitioners, London.

United Kingdom Central Council for Nursing, Midwifery and Health Visiting (1990) *Statement on practice nurses and aspects of the new GP contract* HMSO, London.

Wade, B. (1994) *The Changing Face of Community Care*. Royal College of Nursing, London.

Wallace, P. (1990) Linking up with the over 75s, *British Journal of General Practice*, 4, 267–69.

Williams, E.I & Wallace, P. (1993) *Health Checks for People Aged 75 and Over*. Occasional paper 59. Royal College of General Practitioners, London.

Williamson, J. (1981) Screening, surveillance and case-finding, in *Health Care of the Elderly*. (Ed. by T. Arie) Croom Helm, London.

12.8 APPENDIX: HEALTH CHECKS FOR PEOPLE AGED 75 AND OVER. SOURCE: *JOURNAL OF THE ROYAL COLLEGE OF GENERAL PRACTITIONERS, OCCASIONAL PAPER 59*

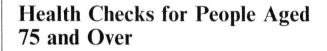

OCCASIONAL PAPER **59**

Health Checks for People Aged 75 and Over

E IDRIS WILLIAMS, MD, FRCGP
Professor of General Practice
University of Nottingham

PAUL WALLACE, MSc, MRCGP
Professor of Primary Health Care
Royal Free Hospital School of Medicine
London

Published by
The Royal College of General Practitioners

April 1993

APPENDIX 1

Health checks for people aged 75 and over

STAGE 1

Health check schedule

The stage 1 health check schedule is intended to be used by any appropriately trained health care professional. It can be used in the person's home and/or opportunistically at the surgery.

The schedule has been developed on the basis of previous work with screening programmes and has been piloted in the Kensington, Chelsea and Westminster Family Health Services Authority area. It is being more extensively evaluated as part of a major multi-centre randomized controlled trial carried out under the auspices of the Medical Research Council.

The health check sheets should be used as a guide to the questions asked and the information obtained recorded on a summary card. It is recommended that this be filled in as each section is completed.

There are 10 sections in all, each containing a set of questions designed to identify problems which should trigger further assessment. The stage 2 primary care assessment schedule sets out the recommended further primary care assessments in sections which correspond to the stage 1 health check.

SOCIAL ASSESSMENT

1. Does someone else live at home with you?
.... If **Yes**

2. Do you generally look after him/her (I mean help to wash, dress, get around)?
                                                                                 Yes**
.... If **No**

3. Do you see relatives, friends or neighbours at least two or three times a week?
.... No*

4. Do you have a relative, neighbour or friend who you can call on for help when required?
.... No*

*Further social assessment indicated (see page 13)
**Further carer and social assessment indicated (see pages 13–14)

HOME ENVIRONMENT

1. In the last year, have you had difficulty keeping your home warm?
.... Yes*

2. In the last 6 months have you had any falls at home?
.... Yes*

3. Is there anything about your home that needs changing?
.... Yes*

   Independent of subject's view, do you believe there is anything about his/her home environment that needs modification?
.... Yes*

*Further home assessment indicated (see page 14)

MOBILITY

Do you, or could you if you had to:

1. Go up and down stairs and steps on your own (if necessary using a frame, tripod or stick)?
.... No*

2. Walk 50 yards down the road on your own (if necessary using a frame, tripod or stick)?
.... No*

*Further functional and home assessment indicated (see pages 14–15)

GENERAL FUNCTION

Do you, or could you if you had to:

1. Do the shopping by yourself?
....No*

2. Do light housework or simple repairs by yourself?
....No*

3. Cook a hot meal by yourself?
....No*

4. Cut your own toenails?
....No*

5. Wash all over on your own (including bathing or showering)?
....No*

6. Dress yourself including zips and buttons?
....No*

*Further functional/physical and home assessment indicated (see pages 14–15)

SENSES

1. Do you have any difficulties hearing and understanding what a person says to you (even if you are wearing a hearing aid) in a quiet room if they speak normally to you?
....Yes*

2. Do you have any difficulty in seeing newsprint, even when you are wearing your glasses?
....Yes**

*Further hearing assessment indicated (see page 16)
**Further visual assessment indicated (see page 16)

CONTINENCE

1. Do you ever wet yourself if you are not able to get to the toilet as soon as you need to, when asleep, or if you cough or sneeze?
....If **Yes**

2. Does this usually happen at least once a week?
....Yes*

3. Do you ever soil or mess yourself?
....Yes*

*Further continence and home assessment indicated (see pages 14–15)

MEDICATION

1. Do you usually take any medication prescribed by your doctor?
....If **Yes**

2. How many different ones? List:
....
....
....(if > 3*)

3. Do you have difficulty in remembering when to take them?
....If **Yes***

4. Are the medications on repeat prescription?
....If **Yes***

*Further medication review indicated (see page 16)

MENTAL FUNCTION

Some practices may prefer to use the Geriatric Depression Scale and Abbreviated Mental Test Score to assess mental function in stage 1 (see below).

1. Do you feel sad, depressed or miserable?

. . . . Yes*

2. Do you have problems with your everyday memory?

. . . . Yes*

Does the elderly person's attitude or behaviour suggest agitation, depression or mental impairment?

. . . . Yes*

*Further mental assessment indicated (see page 17)

SCREENING QUESTIONNAIRE FOR DEPRESSION
Geriatric Depression Scale (GDS) (shortened form)

• Are you basically satisfied with your life?	yes/**No**
• Have you dropped many of your activities and interests?	**Yes**/no
• Do you feel that your life is empty?	**Yes**/no
• Do you often get bored?	**Yes**/no
• Are you in good spirits most of the time?	yes/**No**
• Are you afraid that something bad is going to happen to you?	**Yes**/no
• Do you feel happy most of the time?	yes/**No**
• Do you often feel helpless?	**Yes**/no
• Do you prefer to stay at home, rather than going out and doing new things?	**Yes**/no
• Do you feel you have more problems with memory than most?	**Yes**/no
• Do you think it is wonderful to be alive now?	yes/**No**
• Do you feel pretty worthless the way you are now?	**Yes**/no
• Do you feel full of energy?	yes/**No**
• Do you feel that your situation is hopeless?	**Yes**/no
• Do you think that most people are better off than you are?	**Yes**/no

For each answer in bold type score 1.   Scores >5 indicate probable depression.

Source: Shelk and Yesavage (1986).   See also Appendix 8.

SCREENING QUESTIONNAIRE FOR COGNITIVE FUNCTION
Abbreviated Mental Test Score (AMTS)

May I ask you some routine questions to gauge your memory?

• How old are you?

• What is the time (to nearest hour)?

• Give the patient the following address to recall at end of test: 42 West Street. This should be repeated by the patient to ensure it has been heard correctly.

• What year is it?

• What is your address?

• What jobs do these people do? (Show the patient two pictures: a postman or a cook.) *or* Who are these two people? (Show photographs of Pope and Queen)

• What is your date of birth?

• What year did the First World War start?

• What is the name of the present monarch?

• Please count backwards from 20 to 1.

Then don't forget the address for recall.

Score 1 only for each correct answer.   0–3 indicates severe impairment. 4–6 moderate impairment. >6 is normal.

Source: Hodgkinson HM (1972).   See also Appendix 9.

FINANCES

1. Do you have any difficulty in making ends meet, I mean is it difficult to find the money to pay your bills?
   . . . . Yes*

2. Do you have any difficulty in managing your own finances, I mean things like paying for bills, working out change, etc?
   . . . . Yes*

*See Appendix 4 and possibly refer to Department of Social Security.

LIFESTYLE

1. In general, how often do you have a drink of alcohol?
   . . . . Every day*

2. Do you smoke cigarettes?
   . . . . If **Yes**

   About how many do you usually smoke?
   . . . . [> 20]*

*Further lifestyle review indicated (see page 17)

APPENDIX 8

Geriatric Depression Scale (GDS)

Instructions:

1. Please ask the patient all of the following questions. Ask him/her to choose the best answer for how he/she has felt over the last week.

2. Scoring: Record the patient's response by circling either Yes/No for each question. Total the score obtained when the assessment is complete.

		Yes	No
1.	Are you basically satisfied with your life?	0	1
2.	Have you dropped many of your activities and interests?	1	0
3.	Do you feel that your life is empty?	1	0
4.	Do you often get bored?	1	0
5.	Are you in good spirits most of the time?	0	1
6.	Are you afraid that something bad is going to happen to you?	1	0
7.	Do you feel happy most of the time?	0	1
8.	Do you often feel helpless?	1	0
9.	Do you prefer to stay at home rather than going out and doing new things?	1	0
10.	Do you feel you have more problems with your memory than most?	1	0
11.	Do you think it is wonderful to be alive now?	0	1
12.	Do you feel pretty worthless the way you are now?	1	0
13.	Do you feel full of energy?	0	1
14.	Do you feel that your situation is hopeless?	1	0
15.	Do you think that most people are better off than you are?	1	0

Total score   / 15

A score of > 5 indicates probable depression.

Source: Shelk JI and Yesavage JA (1986) Geriatric Depression Scale (GDS): recent evidence and development of a shorter version. In Brink TL (ed) *Clinical Gerontology: A Guide to Assessment and Intervention.* New York, Haworth Press.

APPENDIX 9

Abbreviated Mental Test Score (AMTS)

Instructions:

1. Please ask the patient all of the following questions.

2. Scoring: A score of 1 is obtained for every correct answer given by the patient.
   When assessment is complete, total the score.

Score

1. How old are you?

2. What time is it (to nearest hour)?

3. Give the patient the following address for recall at end of test:

   42 West Street

   This should be repeated by the patient to ensure it has been heard correctly.

4. What year is it?

5. What is your address?

6. What jobs do these people do? (Show the patient two pictures: a postman and a cook) *or*
   Who are these two people? (Show pictures of Pope and Queen.)

7. What is your date of birth?

8. What year did the First World War start?

9. What is the name of the present monarch?

10. Count backwards from 20–1.

    DON'T FORGET THE ADDRESS FOR RECALL!

    Total Score   / 10

    0–3   Severe impairment

    4–6   Moderate impairment

    > 6   Normal

Source: Hodgkinson HM (1972) Evaluation of a mental test score for assessment of mental impairment in the elderly.
Age and Ageing 1, 233–8.

13

Stroke Rehabilitation
Bernard Gibbon

13.1 INTRODUCTION

Stroke is characterised as

'a focal neurological deficit due to local disturbance in the blood supply to the brain: its onset is usually abrupt, but it may extend over a few hours or longer ... it persists for more than 24 hours'
(World Health Organisation 1971)

An average health district with a population of 250 000 expects to have about 500–650 new stroke patients per year and to have about 900–1200 stroke survivors with some degree of disability living within its boundaries (Wade, 1989). There is some evidence that the incidence of stroke is declining (Dombovey et al., 1986) and this decline continues to be a target for action as detailed in the Government paper The Health of the Nation (Department of Health, 1992). The prevalence of stroke, however, has increased and serves to enhance the emphasis that must be placed on rehabilitation.

Although stroke can occur at any age, the incidence increases with age and approximately 80% of stroke patients are aged over 65 years with men and women being equally affected. Stroke is the third most common cause of death in the UK.

The care of patients following stroke is a common problem encountered by nurses in both hospital and community settings, with roughly equal proportions of people suffering a stroke being admitted to hospital and cared for at home. Studies have shown that about 20% of all medical beds are occupied by stroke patients and the cost of this is estimated to be about 5% of the hospital budget for acute care (Wade et al., 1985).

13.2 PATHOLOGY OF STROKE

The blood supply to the brain is via the carotid arteries which originate from the aorta soon after it leaves the left ventricle of the heart. The carotid arteries divide into the internal and external carotids. The external carotid arteries supply the face and scalp whereas the internal carotid arteries ascend to form the Circle of Willis with the basilar artery which derives from the vertebral arteries. The Circle of Willis supplies blood to the cerebral arteries which supply the brain. There are 3 pairs of cerebral arteries, anterior, middle and posterior (Fig. 13.1).

Areas of the brain have specific functions. For example, the frontal lobes are concerned with personality and the most posterior part concerned with motor activity, the parietal lobe is primarily concerned with appreciation of sensation, the occipital lobe is concerned with vision and the temporal lobe is concerned with taste, sound and smell.

The anterior cerebral artery supplies blood to most of the frontal lobe and the middle cerebral artery supplies the rest of the frontal region and the temporal and parietal lobes. The posterior cerebral arteries supply the occipital lobe. The sensory and motor areas of the brain are therefore supplied blood largely by the middle cerebral artery.

13.4 GUIDANCE FOR PRACTICE – MANAGEMENT OF ACUTE STROKE

Position

Those people who are unconscious or drowsy following stroke will require appropriate positioning to maintain their airway and prevent naso-pharyngeal secretions entering the respiratory system. The person should be positioned in either the lateral or semi-prone position and maintained in this position by the use of pillows. Patients who have lost their swallow reflex are at risk of aspirating naso-pharyngeal secretions and subsequently contracting chest infections.

Skin

Skin integrity is at risk if the patient is maintained in one position too long and the appropriate use of a pressure sore risk assessment tool, for example the Waterlow Scale (Waterlow 1985), should be used in conjunction with a turning protocol. The Lowthian Turning Chart (Lowthian, 1985), modified to exclude prone lying which may increase muscle tone in the stroke patient, will reduce the risk of pressure sore development. In addition to positioning, the patient must be handled carefully to prevent damage to joints, especially on the affected side and to prevent skin damage secondary to friction or dragging. (See also Chapter 5.)

Nutrition and hydration

An adequate state of hydration and nutrition will reduce the risk of pressure sore development as well as maintaining the general health of the patient. A daily intake of approximately 2 litres of fluid is necessary and an intravenous infusion may be required if the patient cannot tolerate fluids orally. It is important to undertake a swallowing assessment prior to introducing oral drinking and feeding to ensure there is no risk of aspiration. It should be remembered that fluids are more easily aspirated than foods and that a gag reflex does not necessarily indicate that a swallow is normal. Swallowing assessments may be undertaken by speech and language therapists

and the local hospital department will be able to provide information on the service. Introducing a naso-gastric tube may lead to oesophagitis and inhibit the return of the swallowing reflex.

Remembering to position the patient upright during, and for half an hour after eating and drinking may overcome many difficulties. Thickening foods and fluids with commercially available thickening powders may also help. Protracted swallowing problems leading to nutritional deficit can be addressed by insertion of a percutaneous endoscopic gastrostomy feeding tube. Nutritionally deficient patients are not best placed to participate in active rehabilitation activities. (See also Chapter 3.)

Elimination

A major contribution of nursing care to the stroke patient is the management of elimination. Urinary incontinence may be managed in the short term by frequent changes and attention to hygiene but catheterisation may be necessary if there is a risk to the integument. Retention of urine will require the insertion of a catheter, but a self retaining catheter may not be essential unless the problem recurs. Patients who lose continence following a stroke and subsequently regain continence frequently make a substantial recovery and as such this acts as an optimistic prognostic indicator (Barer, 1989).

Faecal elimination also requires careful management as constipation may lead to an increase in muscle tone and increases the risk of spasticity. (See also Chapter 8.)

13.5 GUIDANCE FOR PRACTICE – PATIENT ASSESSMENT

A comprehensive assessment must be undertaken in order to determine the individual patient's care and rehabilitation needs (Andrews & Stewart, 1979). The use of an appropriate assessment tool is often helpful in ensuring that all relevant data have been collected.

Relevant data must also include an assessment of the patient's pre-stroke health status, in particular mental status, mobility and continence, together with details of general living conditions. This provides useful data upon which to plan care.

Table 13.1 The Barthel Index. Source: *Maryland State Medical Journal*, 14, 61–5, Mahoney, F.I. & Barthel, D.W. (1965), Functional evaluation: the Barthel Index.

	Score
Bowels	
Incontinent (or needs enema)	0
Occasional accident	1
Continent	2
Bladder	
Incontinent	0
Occasional accident	1
Continent	2
Grooming	
Needs help	0
Independent for face/hair/teeth/shaving	1
Toilet use	
Dependent	0
Needs some help but can do some alone	1
Independent in all actions	2
Feeding	
Dependent	0
Needs some help, e.g. cutting, but can feed self	1
Independent in all actions	2
Transfer bed–chair and back	
Dependent, can't sit	0
Needs major help (2 people), can sit	1
Minor help (1 person) or supervision	2
Independent	3
Mobility	
Immobile	0
Independent in wheelchair	1
Walks with help of 1 or supervision	2
Walks independently (+/– aid)	3
Dressing	
Dependent	0
Needs help, does half	1
Independent (includes buttons, zips, laces)	2
Stairs	
Unable to manage	0
Needs to help	1
Independent	2
Bathing	
Dependent	0
Independent (or in shower)	1
Total	

Assessment is an on-going activity and the individual stroke patient's progress can be measured using activities of daily living (ADL) scales such as the Barthel Index (see Table 13.1) which provide an objective means of measuring progress (Gibbon, 1991).

An assessment of the current health status is also a necessary pre-requisite of rehabilitation planning. Problem identification, should be prioritised according to problems which are life threatening, those that threaten to change a person destructively and problems that affect the person's normal growth and development.

Care plans are frequently discipline specific with reference to other disciplines featuring only as a referral entry. In situations where several members of the multidisciplinary team are involved simultaneously with the care, management and rehabilitation of the patient a collaborative care plan is most beneficial. The collaborative care plan ensures coordination of effort and the resolution of conflicting goals. Additionally it places the patient at the centre of the interventions rather than as a recipient of the professionals' objectives. In the community, for example, the GP, community nurse and day hospital may all be involved in the management of a patient.

The common physical problems associated with stroke are loss of consciousness or drowsiness, hemiplegia, difficulty with balance and mobility, dysphagia, dysphasia, and incontinence of urine. Psychologically the patient may have disturbance to memory (loss of both short term and long term), perceptual problems, depression, and emotional lability. Social problems include feelings of isolation, change in role(s), financial and work concerns (Gibbon, 1994a).

The aims of nursing management in the acute phase are to sustain life and prevent complications occurring. Complications of stroke include:

■ Deep vein thrombosis
■ Pneumonia
■ Pressure sores
■ Urinary tract infections
■ Joint contractures
■ Shoulder pain/dislocation
■ Depression.

Skilful nursing intervention not only sustains life but ensures that the rehabilitative aspects of care com-

mence immediately and are sustained throughout the patient's recovery.

13.6 GUIDANCE FOR PRACTICE – REHABILITATION

Rehabilitation can be defined as:

'restoring the abilities and functions of an individual to a prior level in social, physical, emotional and economic spheres.'   (Baroch 1976)

The aim of rehabilitation is toward restoration of self care abilities and the reduction of dependence. Rehabilitation, as a legitimate activity of nursing, does not appear to have universal acceptance amongst the profession and reasons for this are not clear (Gibbon & Thompson, 1992; Gibbon, 1994b). To some extent the problem seems to arise out of difficulty in defining the role of the nurse in general, let alone in rehabilitation. For example, rehabilitation of post myocardial infarction patients appears to be accepted as nursing's role but stroke rehabilitation, perhaps because of the perceived requirement for special techniques, seems to be passed almost entirely into the therapist's domain (Gibbon, 1994b). This has led some to the conclusion that nurses lack the confidence and skills to be autonomous in rehabilitation interventions (Myco, 1984).

In a hospital context, Waters (1991) suggested that nurses acted as understudies for therapists and largely only became involved in rehabilitation activities when they needed to 'stand in' for therapists at weekends and evenings. O'Connor (1993) also suggested that the role of the nurse was to be supportive to therapists. The autonomous role of the nurse in stroke rehabilitation still requires clarification. Promoting self care and independence appears to be a concept with which community nurses are comfortable, and in relation to the stroke patient can be regarded as synonymous with rehabilitation.

Aims of rehabilitation

The aims of rehabilitative interventions in stroke care are to:

- prevent deformities;
- facilitate motor recovery;
- facilitate functional recovery in activities of daily living;
- motivate the patient towards self care and independence;
- promote psychosocial integration.

Principles of rehabilitation

Newman (1985) suggested that three basic principles underpin stroke rehabilitation:

(1) If one side of the brain is injured, the opposite side of the body will be affected.
(2) Specific centres of the brain control particular body functions and the effects of the stroke will depend on the site and size of the lesion.
(3) The maximum traumatic effect of the stroke will occur several hours after the onset, due to increasing oedema of the surrounding tissue. The disability of survivors will gradually lessen as the oedema reduces.

Pattern of recovery

A typical pattern of recovery has been identified in hemiplegic stroke patients. Recovery of leg function occurs before arm function, and arm function prior to hand function and this will influence the activation programme. Appropriate interventions commencing in the immediate post stroke period have been demonstrated to have a beneficial effect on the degree of recovery following stroke.

Prevention of deformities

To prevent deformities and joint contractures occurring the patient should be nursed in the correct position. This may be conceptualised as a position that opposes the direction of flexion.

The importance of exercises – passive, assisted or active – and early weight bearing are also important to contracture prevention and the entire health care team including informal carers must take responsibility for ensuring that therapy continues.

Psychosocial rehabilitation

Promoting psychosocial rehabilitation must not be ignored in favour of functional recovery. Changes to mood states and emotionalism are common sequelae to stroke (House *et al.*, 1989) and may act as a barrier to successful rehabilitation unless adequately addressed. These changes can be particularly distressing to family members. Activities such as engaging the patient in conversation purposefully, frequently and regularly, perhaps with conversation relating to the 'here and now,' act as stimuli. Encouraging the patient to participate in social activities ranging from joining others whilst eating through to organised events can be rewarding to the patient and family alike.

Teamwork

Care planning should be based on the principles of SMART planning, that is goals should be Specific, Measurable, Achievable, Realistic and Time stated. The most effective goals in maximising the patient's potential are considered to be those that lead to reward and reinforcement of behaviour, those that are short term and realistic, and those which involve not only patients and their families, but also other members of the health care team.

The rehabilitation team (taken to include the family/carer) must work as an interdisciplinary team, with patient-centred goals as the focus of care. This approach ensures consistency and continuity of care with each occupational group accepting that grey areas exist between the expertise associated with the different disciplines. The importance of patient- and carer-centred goals over a professional group's objectives cannot be overstated.

Conflict and petty jealousies have been reported between occupational groups when understanding has been found wanting (Spiby, 1988) and these are considered to have impeded developments in rehabilitation. Fragmentation of care must be avoided and mutual respect fostered within the team. Nurses usually have the most day-to-day contact with stroke patients and are increasingly assuming the role of key worker or care manager for this group. It follows therefore that nurses need to have a clear understanding not only of the individual care plan but of the principles and practice of rehabilitation.

13.7 GUIDANCE FOR PRACTICE – REHABILITATION TECHNIQUES

Positioning the stroke patient

Stroke patients typically adopt a position in which the affected arm is held close to the body with the elbow and wrist in a flexed (bent) position and the fingers and thumb flexed to form a 'claw like' hand. The lower limb is also held in flexion. If the patient is allowed to remain in this position many complications will arise, such as, contractures, development of pressure sores and respiratory difficulty as well as discomfort. Contractures are painful, disfiguring and prevent the person regaining independence in the activities of daily living. Once contractures have developed they cannot be reversed.

The aim is to reduce spasticity and contractures by maintaining reflex inhibiting patterns of posture and the key to correct positioning is a normal or neutral posture (Fig. 13.2). The head and neck should be supported in a symmetrical position when the patient is sitting and additionally, if lying on the affected side, the head should be placed forward. Supine lying should be avoided if possible but the head should be centrally placed and slightly forward if adopted.

Care of the upper limb involves positioning in which the shoulder should be protracted with the arm brought forward:

- to 90° to body when lying on affected side;
- supported on pillows to level when lying on unaffected side;
- positioned symmetrically on lap pillow when sitting, elbow flexed (*not* allowed to hang down);
- with the wrist maintained in a neutral position;
- with the hand pronated (palm downwards);
- with the fingers extended.

The body or trunk of the person should be straight and mid-line and flexion of the trunk should be avoided. Whilst in the lying position the back should be at 90° to the bed and pillows will often have to be used to maintain the position.

Care of the lower limb involves the following actions:

- The knee should be flexed in the side lying posi-

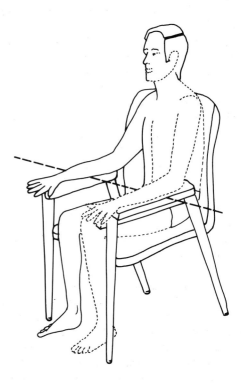

Figure 13.2 Correct positioning of the patient (the paralysed side of the body is indicated by the broken line). Source: *The Stroke Patient: A Team Approach* (3rd edn) by M. Johnstone, courtesy of Churchill Livingstone.

tion and be forward with support from a pillow when lying on the unaffected side.
- Both legs should be straight out in front when sitting in bed.
- The hip, knee and ankle should be flexed at right angles (90°).

Physiotherapy

This has been regarded as the mainstay of therapy for stroke patients (University of Leeds *et al.*, 1992). Physiotherapy is now more readily available in the community where fundholding GPs have employed physiotherapists on a sessional basis. The Bobath Technique is commonly adopted and this seeks to exploit the untapped potential of the affected side of the brain by inhibition of abnormal patterns of spasticity and by the facilitation and stimulation of normal autonomic and voluntary functional movements (Bobath, 1978).

The person can be conceptualised as being an adaptive organism which learns through experience and exposure to environmental stimuli and this is particularly evident in the central nervous system which is a response-based system. The physiotherapist will conduct an assessment to determine the patient's main problems and a treatment plan is worked out to address these problems. Normal movement, like normal positioning, is the basis for the physiotherapy treatment of stroke patients.

The nurse has a responsibility to be aware of the therapy plan and to assist with its implementation. Whilst sitting, the patient should be seated well back in the chair and look symmetrical, not being allowed to slump to one side. This position, by supporting the lumbar spine, prevents it becoming flexed.

Both arms should be placed in front of the patient on a pillow on the lap and the affected arm should not be allowed to dangle over the arm of the chair. This provides support for the shoulder and allows the patient to see and acknowledge both arms. If the arm is flaccid it is vitally important to protect the shoulder. The lack of muscle tone means that there is no resistance to overstretching and a subluxation (dislocation) may easily occur. The shoulder should be handled carefully during all transfers and also when the patient is being positioned in bed. Any movement which involves overstretch or distraction of the joint should be avoided (Wood, 1989).

Occupational therapy

Occupational therapy which aims to assist the patient to return to the fullest possible physical, psychological and social recovery (Nicholls, 1980) is also the mainstay of therapy for stroke patients. The occupational therapist, like the physiotherapist, will undertake an assessment of the patient and the nurse must share the therapist's goals to assist in the rehabilitation process. Frequently the physiotherapist and occupational therapist work closely together, especially in the hospital setting, but this is not always the case in the community.

The occupational therapist undertakes home assessments to determine the patient's functional ability and encourages maximum independence in activities of daily living, which may include the provision of equipment (e.g. adapted cutlery) or teaching a new technique (e.g. getting dressed whilst sitting).

It is important for community nurses to liaise with the therapists, at the case conference, ward round or informally in order that they can fully contribute to the therapeutic process.

Speech and language therapy

Whilst there is no doubting the expertise of the speech and language therapist in treating patients with communication and swallowing difficulties, there are a number of practical actions that a nurse can undertake. Communication difficulties or dysphasias can be classified as either receptive, difficulty in understanding, or expressive, difficulty in expressing or articulating words.

Patients with difficulty in understanding (receptive dysphasia) often follow the gist of a message by using non-verbal behaviours and it may be useful to face the person directly and use short sentences emphasising the main words. Speaking slowly and clearly with background noise kept to a minimum is also recommended.

People with expressive dysphasia frequently get frustrated at their inability to make others understand and it is important to remain relaxed and not give patients the impression of impatience with them. Encouraging patients who cannot express words to use alternative means, for example, writing, gesture or drawing, may provide an appropriate channel of communication and alleviate frustration. It should be noted that 'Yes/No' answers are often confused in both expressive and receptive dysphasia.

In essence, when communicating with a dysphasic person it is important to be a good listener and provide feedback to the person. It is as important for the person to know whether they have been understood or not.

Dysphagia management

Dysphagia management frequently requires assessment by a speech and language therapist and subsequent intervention planning. A number of signs may indicate swallowing problems including weight loss and chest infections as well as drooling, coughing (before, during or after swallowing) and pocketing of food in the mouth.

The management of swallowing difficulties will include only giving food/drink when the patient is sitting upright with the head supported as necessary. The patient should be kept upright for at least 30 minutes after eating or drinking and only small amounts or sips of fluid should be given. Following eating the mouth should be checked for pocketed food.

Clinical investigations

Clinical examination frequently confirms the diagnosis of stroke and extensive investigations are not usually warranted. The aim of investigations is to find a cause for the stroke and where possible treat an identified cause. Blood pressure measurement will be undertaken but blood pressure is usually elevated following stroke and this should not be treated with hypotensive agents as this may exacerbate the cerebral damage.

Other investigations would include:

- Blood glucose estimation to determine the presence of diabetes and cholesterol levels to detect the presence of hyperlipidaemia.
- Erythrocyte sedimentation rate (ESR) would be undertaken to exclude temporal arteritis as a cause of the stroke.
- X-ray of the chest and skull may be undertaken to exclude tumours as the cause.
- A skull X-ray may also show a sub-dural haematoma as a possible cause of the stroke.
- A lumbar puncture may be undertaken to exclude meningitis.

More recently, investigations such as CT (computer tomography) scanning have been undertaken. These have the advantage of being relatively simple, quick, non-invasive and accurate, but they do not provide evidence about the extent of the cerebral infarction until several days after the acute onset (Wester *et al.*, 1992).

Monitoring progress

Measurement tools have long been established to quantify aspects of patient care, including those relating to stroke. Such indicators generally measure impairment, the physiological consequences of pathology, disability, the functional consequences and handicap, the social consequences.

Disability is considered to be the central focus of recovery following stroke and a number of 'tools' have been devised to measure the functional recovery of the patient, usually based on activities of daily living (Gibbon, 1991).

A widely accepted tool which studies have shown to be valid and reliable is the Barthel Index (Mahoney & Barthel 1965) (Table 13.1); and Wade (1988) cautions against the development of more and more tools which have use only to those who devise them. Despite criticism of the Barthel Index, usually of its lack of sensitivity to individual patients, it remains one of the most widely used tools in measuring functional recovery following stroke. The domains assessed in the Barthel Index include functional independence in bowel and bladder control, grooming and dressing, eating and drinking, transferring, mobility including stairs, and bathing.

13.8 SUMMARY

Stroke is the third most common cause of death in the UK; an average health district has about 900–1200 stroke survivors with some degree of disability living within its boundaries (Wade, 1989). The community nurse is commonly involved in the care of patients following stroke; the nurse is often a member of a multidisciplinary team involving the patient and family in the rehabilitation process.

There is some controversy in the literature regarding the nurse's role in the rehabilitation process and the role of the community nurse in rehabilitation of patients with stroke requires further clarification. Notwithstanding this community nurses have a key role in providing direct care and family support for this patient group.

13.9 REFERENCES AND FURTHER READING

Andrews, K. & Stewart, J. (1979) Stroke recovery: he can but does he? *Rheumatology and Rehabilitation*, **18**, 43–8.

Barer, D.H. (1989) Continence after stroke, *Age and Ageing*, **18**, 183–91.

Baroch, R.M. (1976) *Elements of Rehabilitation in Nursing*. C.V. Mosby, St Louis.

Barrett, J., Jones, M., Relston, A. & Ayris, G. (1992) Principles of stroke rehabilitation, *Nursing the Elderly*, **4**, 5, 18.

Bobath, B. (1978) *Adult Hemiplegia: Evaluation and Treatment*. William Heinemann, London.

Boore, J.R.P., Champion, R. & Ferguson, M.C. (1987) *Nursing the Physically Ill Adult*. Churchill Livingstone, Edinburgh.

Carr, E.K. & Kenney, F.D. (1992) Positioning of the stroke patient: a review of the literature, *International Journal of Nursing Studies*, **29**, 4, 355–69.

Department of Health (1992) *The Health of the Nation*. Department of Health, London.

Dombovy, M.L., Sandok, B.A. & Basford, J.R. (1986) Rehabilitation for Stroke, *Stroke*, **17**, 3, 363–9.

Gibbon, B. (1991) Measuring Stroke Recovery, *Nursing Times*, **87**, 44, 32–4.

Gibbon, B. (1994a) Stroke care and rehabilitation (Continuing Education Series Paper and Assessment) *Nursing Standard*, **8**, 33, 49–56.

Gibbon, B. (1994b) Stroke nursing care and management in the community: a survey of district nurses' perceived contribution in one health district, *Journal of Advanced Nursing*, **16**, 11, 1136–42.

Gibbon, B. & Thompson, A. (1992) An exploration of nurses' understanding of their role in rehabilitation, *Nursing Standard*, **6**, 36, 32–5.

House, A., Dennis, M., Molyneux, A., Warlow, C. & Hawton, K. (1989) Emotionalism after stroke, *British Medical Journal*, **298**, 991–4.

Lowthian, P. (1985) Preventing pressure sores, *Nursing Mirror*, **160**, 25, 18–20.

Mahoney, F.I. & Barthel, D.W. (1965) Functional evaluation: the Barthel Index, *Maryland State Medical Journal*, **14**, 61–5.

Marmot, M.G. & Poulter, N.R. (1992) Primary prevention of stroke, *The Lancet*, **339**, 344–7.

Mulley, G. & Arie, T. (1978) Treating stroke: hospital or home, *British Medical Journal*, 11 July, 1321–2.

Myco, F. (1983) *Nursing Care of the Hemiplegic Stroke Patient*. Harper and Row, London.

Myco, F. (1984) Stroke and its rehabilitation: the perceived role of the nurse in the medical and nursing literature, *Journal of Advanced Nursing*, **9**, 429–39.

Newman, D. (1985) Essential physical therapy for stroke patients, *Nursing Times*, **81**, 16–18.

Nicholls, P.J.R. (1980) *Rehabilitation Medicine – The Management of Physical Disabilities*. Butterworth, London.

Norton, D., McLaren, R. & Exton-Smith, A.N. (1962) *An Investigation of Geriatric Nursing Problems in Hospital*. National Corporation for the Care of Old People, London.

O'Connor, S.E. (1993) Nursing and rehabilitation: the interventions of nurses in stroke patient care, *Journal of Clinical Nursing*, **2**, 29–34.

Spiby, J. (1988) A stroke of bad luck, *Nursing Times*, **84**, 29, 21.

University of Leeds, University of York, Royal College of Physicians (1992) *Effective Health Care: Stroke Rehabilitation*. University of Leeds, Leeds.

Wade, D.T., Wood, V.A. & Langton-Hewer, R. (1985) Use of hospital resources by acute stroke patients, *Journal of Royal College of Physicians*, **19**, 48–52.

Wade, D.T. & Langton-Hewer, R. (1986) Epidemiology of some neurological diseases with special reference to workload on NHS, *International Rehabilitation Medicine*, **8**, 129–37.

Wade, D.T. (1988) Measurement in rehabilitation, *Age and Ageing*, **17**, 289–92.

Wade, D. (1989) Organisation of stroke care services, *Clinical Rehabilitation*, **3**, 227–33.

Waterlow, J. (1985) A risk assessment card, *Nursing Times*, **81**, 49–55.

Waters, K. (1991) The role of the nurse in the rehabilitation of elderly people in hospital. Unpublished PhD Thesis, University of Manchester.

Wester, P.O., Asplund, K., Eriksson, S., Holm, J., Marke L., Norlund, A., Norrving, B., Normell, L. & Rehncrona (1992) *Stroke*. The Swedish Council on Technology Assessment in Health Care, Stockholm.

Wood, C. (1989) Shoulder pain in stroke patients, *Nursing Times*, **85**, 2, 32–4.

World Health Organisation (1971) *Cerebrovascular Diseases – Prevention, Treatment and Rehabilitation*. Technical Report Series No 469. World Health Organisation, Geneva.

ACKNOWLEDGEMENTS

The author would like to acknowledge the assistance of Claire Heffer (Speech Therapist), Joyce Riley (Physiotherapist) and Helen Wells (Occupational Therapist) at the Royal Liverpool University Hospital in the preparation of this chapter.

14

Management of Long Term Health Problems
Ann-Louise Caress

14.1 INTRODUCTION

Changes in both the nature of disease and the structure of populations in the last 50 years have had a profound impact upon health in Western societies. The numbers of elderly individuals are rising and will continue to rise towards the turn of the century. Improved health care, particularly for neonates and at times of health crisis, has resulted in greater survival rates.

Such changes as these have resulted in an increased prevalence of chronic illness (Anderson & Bury, 1988) and it is estimated that as many as one in ten of the adult population experiences a degree of physical disability (Hermanova, 1985). The nature of chronic illness is such that the bulk of it is necessarily cared for by community nurses (Hasler, 1985) together with input from patients and their families or other carers.

People with chronic illness will have an extended patient career, requiring long term and often extensive contact with health care professionals. This affects the nature of the relationship between patient and professional. Partly this is due to the greater depth of such relationships. However, the relationship is also altered by the life-long experience of patients and their families, which may lead to them becoming expert in the management of their condition. This highlights a major distinction between care of the acutely and chronically ill patient. Care of chronic illness typically involves the patient in self management (Brearley, 1990). This arises from both the cost of long term care and the desire to minimise disruption of the chronically ill individual's lifestyle. Self management in turn has implications for the knowledge required by chronically ill individuals: in order to carry out care, such patients must understand something of the nature of their illness, its symptoms and their implications, and the procedures necessary to manage their condition.

Caring for chronically ill patients, therefore, can be expected to form an increasing proportion of the work of community nurses. The care of such patients will require community nurses to adopt alternatives to the traditional nurse–patient relationship and to learn skills relevant to activities such as patient education.

14.2 LIVING WITH A LONG TERM HEALTH PROBLEM

Social and medical advances in Western societies have served to increase longevity and diminish mortality from many conditions. However, concomitant with this has been a rise in chronic morbidity and its accompanying problems (Anderson & Bury, 1988). In recent years, social scientists and health care professionals have begun to realise that the effects of long term health problems extend beyond the impact of the disease process itself (Locker, 1983; Strauss & Glaser, 1985).

Locker (1983) identifies three essential aspects of the management of long term health problems:

- Medical – controlling symptoms and minimising the physical impact of the condition.
- Cognitive – dealing with the psychological impact of the problem.

■ Practical – managing the treatment programme and dealing with the impact of the problem on activities and physical capabilities.

Psychological consequences of long term health problems

Changes in mood state amongst the physically ill are widely reported (Zigmond & Snaith, 1983), and are especially commonplace amongst those with long term health problems. In some circumstances, these arise as a result of the disease process (e.g. in Alzheimer's disease or renal failure). Commonly, however, they may be attributable to the impact of the disease process on the patient's life.

Psychological problems include: anxiety, especially when the health problem is poorly controlled or the prognosis uncertain; depression; irritability; and loss of self esteem. These appear to be linked with individuals' perceptions about the impact of the condition upon their quality of life. In some circumstances psychological problems may reflect feelings of loss and frustration at imposed physical handicaps. However, an individual's psychological response to a long term health problem may bear little relation to the degree of physical debility to which the problem gives rise (Anderson & Bury, 1988). It is consequently important that health care professionals do not make the assumption that patients with few physical symptoms will have a better psychological response to their problems than a severely physically impaired individual. Indeed, it has been argued that those with more severe physical symptoms may, in fact, sometimes have a better psychological outcome, since they feel legitimately able to adopt the so-called sick role and hence do not feel obliged to maintain a facade of normality (Anderson & Bury, 1988).

Social consequences of long term health problems

The social functioning of many patients with long term health problems is severely impaired. Common areas which are disrupted include:

■ Ability to work
■ Ability to travel or go on holiday
■ Social life.

All of these aspects can severely impair the perceived quality of life of the chronically ill and will in turn reflect upon their psychological status.

Economic impact of long term health problems

Numerous studies have demonstrated the economically disadvantaged position of many patients with long term health problems. They frequently depend upon state benefits which in recent years have fallen behind average earnings.

Various other factors contribute to financial hardship. Most important amongst these is the loss of earning capability; the physical symptoms or treatment regimen in many long term health problems may debar the patient from remaining in or returning to employment. Even when patients are able to work, they often only do so on a part-time basis.

Discrimination amongst employers against those with health problems is widespread. Individuals may fail to secure employment because of their health history, or may find it difficult to move between jobs. Even when the chronically ill secure a job, they may find themselves passed over for promotion or selected out for redundancy if they have had to have a lot of time off work either as a result of ill-health or of its treatment. Again, it should be noted that it may be the perception of a problem in the mind of an employer, or prospective employer, rather than its actual magnitude which can cause difficulties for the chronically ill.

A further cause of lost income is the frequent need for partners to reduce or even cease their employment in order to care for the patient. Thus it is often the case that more than one of the incomes in a household may be affected by chronic illness.

Finally, there is the cost of treatment itself. Although in the United Kingdom the vast majority of such costs are met by the state, it is still often the case that treatment leaves individuals 'out of pocket'. This is especially the case when the regimen calls for a special diet.

A common feature of long term health problems is a lack of spontaneity. It becomes difficult for patients to do anything or go anywhere without needing to plan and act in advance. Many report that the intrusiveness of their condition is the main factor in its effect upon their life satisfaction.

Effect of long term health problems on the family

The thrust of government health policy in recent years has been towards increasing the amount of care for the chronically ill which is received in the community. In practice, this often means an increased level of input by informal carers, such as family, friends and neighbours – and, by extrapolation, by women (Anderson & Bury, 1988). Long term health problems affect families and carers as much as, and sometimes more than, the patients themselves:

Physical effects
Firstly, there is the physical impact of looking after someone with a long term health problem. Tiredness and fatigue are widely reported amongst carers.

Psychological effects
Long term health problems also have psychological effects upon carers; depression is widely reported, and believed to be underestimated. A common contributor to the problems of carers is the need to cope with mood state and behavioural changes in the person for whom they are caring. A further problem lies in coming to terms with the changes which will have occurred in the person for whom they are caring, for example, in the case of neurological disorders, where a previously active person may become physically dependent. Concomitant with this is the disturbing effect of uncertainty upon the carer. Again neurological conditions serve as a good example: the uncertainty about the degree and severity of physical disability is often reported as a problem amongst carers. The disruption of the carer's social life and lack of spontaneity are also widely commented upon, as is uncertainty about the outcome of illness.

Family roles
The presence of a long term health problem may necessitate a change in roles in a family. A spouse or child may be required to undertake new tasks and responsibilities, e.g. housework, shopping, etc. If the patient ceases to be the main earner in a household, it may require another member of the family to become the main earner. Equally, it may necessitate a carer giving up work. Some long term problems require carers to undertake intimate physical care.

Compliance

The traditional image of the patient–carer relation-ship views the patient as a passive recipient of care, who receives instruction and prescriptions from health care professionals and carries these out undeviatingly and unquestioningly. This view has been widely attacked and challenged in recent years as being unacceptable and unduly simplistic (Brearley, 1990).

It is widely acknowledged that many patients do not follow their prescribed regimen (Sackett & Haynes, 1976; Becker & Maiman, 1975). Previously this was viewed in a negative light, often from a medical standpoint. More recent research has sought to explain so-called non-compliance from the patient's perspective. Psychological and sociological theories have enlightened this exploration, in particular work which examines health beliefs (Becker & Maiman, 1975); concepts of control (Ley, 1982); and the patient–provider relationship (Linn *et al.*, 1982; Feely & Pullar, 1989, Stimson, 1974).

Failure to follow the prescribed regimen may be the result of many factors:

- Denial of the health problem.
- Lack of belief in the effectiveness of the regimen.
- Unacceptable behaviour change required by regimen.
- Unpleasant physical symptoms or side effects from treatment.
- Attempts to minimise impact of the problem on life.
- Attempts to retain control over health and life.
- Conflict between patient and/or carers and health care providers.
- Lack of understanding of or knowledge about the condition or its treatment.
- Prior expectations or misconceptions about the condition and its treatment.

Current approaches aim to explain the causes of patients behaviour, to try to understand how regimens affect their lives and to minimise unacceptable disruption of patients' lifestyles.

Patient education is often viewed as a panacea for non-compliance. However, research suggests that improvements in knowledge will not necessarily be translated into changes in behaviour (Luker & Caress, 1989; Feely & Pullar, 1989), and that relying on supplying or re-stating information to patients who alter their treatment regimen will be insufficient.

Self-management of long term health problems

inevitably means that the patient ceases to be passive in the treatment programme. It must therefore be anticipated that the patient with long term problems will make judgements about the condition, its symptoms and their control and will weigh the costs and benefits of a proposed regimen when deciding whether or not to follow professional advice.

Important points for health care professionals to consider are:

- understanding the patient's perspective;
- minimising negative effects of treatment;
- ensuring consistency of instructions and advice;
- identifying the causes of deviation from the prescribed regimen;
- attempting to avoid employing a punitive response to deviations from the prescribed regimen.

14.3 PRINCIPLES OF PATIENT EDUCATION

Patient education is an important and appropriate nursing activity. The volume of literature on the subject is extensive, with many texts exhorting nurses to undertake patient education (Bille, 1981; Redman, 1981). The process of patient education is typically assumed to be a simple one, yet research evidence indicates that this is not the case.

There is an assumption that mainstream educational principles can be taken and directly applied to patient education. Luker and Caress (1989) argue that this is not, in fact, the case, since the physical and psychological consequences of ill-health can affect the learning process and thus render teaching more difficult.

In addition there also appears to be an assumption that nurses are equipped with the skills necessary to teach. This fails to recognise the complexity of teaching and runs counter to the research which suggests that nurses do not feel adequately prepared to take on the role of teacher (Close, 1988; Tilley *et al.*, 1987).

Finally, the influence of organisational considerations concerning such factors as availability of staff time are neglected in much of the patient education literature.

The term 'patient education' has no single definition. As Wilson-Barnett (1988) points out, for some 'patient education' means little more than information giving. Thus it would encompass only such activities as providing patients with leaflets and booklets.

In the context of chronic care, however, this is typically seen as too limited a definition (Luker & Caress, 1989; Wilson-Barnett, 1988), not least because it must often encompass such activities as instruction in practical procedures and advice about self-management for both patients and their carers. Patient education can be separated into three discrete elements:

- Teaching – which encompasses information-giving and instruction in, for example, performance of procedures.
- Education – which is a more complex undertaking, more interactive and less didactic than teaching.
- Support – which is primarily supporting patients in their independent management of their condition and acting as resource person.

Definition of learning

In order to demonstrate that an intervention has been effective, it is necessary to look at the outcome of the intervention. In the case of teaching, the appropriate outcome is learning. Honey and Mumford (1982) state that learning may be considered to have taken place when people know something they did not know before and can demonstrate this, and when people are able to do something which they could not do before.

Components of learning

Learning theorists have identified three psychological components of learning (Honey & Mumford, 1982). These are:

- Cognition – which concerns an individual's academic ability, alertness, state of orientation, memory, and understanding of material.
- Perception – which concerns an individual's vision, hearing and manual dexterity.
- Affect – which concerns an individual's mood state, motivation and beliefs about the benefits of the learning experience.

The influence of each of these areas must be borne in mind when an educational venture is undertaken. Thus, the most thoroughly prepared educational material will have little impact if the learner is poorly motivated or does not see the relevance of the learning experience. Similarly, attempts to educate an individual who is extremely anxious are unlikely to succeed, since the learner's retention of information will be impaired.

Table 14.1 Kolb's types of learner.

Type descriptor	Preferred method of learning
Accommodator	Concrete experience and active involvement
Converger	Abstract situations and active involvement
Assimilator	Abstract situations and reflection
Diverger	Concrete experience and reflection

Stages of learning

Kolb (1976) has identified four stages of learning, through which all individuals pass when exposed to novel information or situations:

- Concrete experience – involvement in new experiences.
- Reflective observation – reflection and pondering on experience.
- Abstract conceptualisation – formulation of theories and hypotheses based on experience.
- Active experimentation – testing of these hypotheses.

It is important to recognise the stage which the learner is presently at when educating individuals, since this will affect the type of intervention which it is appropriate to employ. For example, following a new experience, time should be allowed for the individual to reflect upon it before moving on to new material. Similarly, after a new experience, the teacher should anticipate the learner developing hypotheses and needing to ask questions which affirm or refute these. Consequently, time must be planned into a teaching schedule to enable the educator to be available for answering questions.

Types of learner

Based on the identification of stages of learning, Kolb (1976) also details four types of learner (Table 14.1). These types involve combinations of those who prefer concrete experience (seeing it for real) versus abstract situations (watching, listening, theoretical problems), and active involvement ('hands on') versus reflection ('in your head').

Matching the learning experience to the type of learner can result in improved learning outcome. However, this assumes some prior assessment of learning capabilities and preferences, and an ability on the part of the educator to undertake such assessment.

Teaching styles

Learning is dependent not only upon the learner, but also upon the quality of the educational experience. The concept of androgogy refers to the idea that adults have different learning needs from children (Kidd, 1973). It is argued that adults learn best through experiential learning, an educational method championed by Boydell (1985). This method advocates drawing upon prior life experience to inform teaching and using 'real-life' situations. Brookfield (1986) suggests that adult learning can be enhanced by paying attention to the following factors:

- The learning situation should be learner rather than teacher centred, i.e. directed by the learner's educational needs.
- Learning should be autonomous, rather than directed, allowing the learner to set the pace and direction of the learning.
- Active involvement in learning is preferable to the

learner being passive. This does not necessarily mean providing concrete experience, but means engaging the learner, rather than simply preaching to them.

■ Meaningful learning results in an improved outcome over rote learning. Consequently, teaching should have relevance to the individual's life experience and present situation.

14.4 GUIDANCE FOR PRACTICE – PATIENT EDUCATION

Consideration when presenting material

In order for teaching material to be well received by the learner, a number of considerations about its presentation must be borne in mind (Doak *et al.*, 1986):

■ Teach the smallest amount possible.
■ Make the point as vividly as possible.
■ Review material repeatedly.
■ Have the learner re-state and demonstrate material.

Problems in patient education

The process of patient education may be complicated by a number of factors (Luker & Caress, 1989). These may be divided into three areas:

■ Patient related factors
■ Nurse related factors
■ Organisational factors

Patient related factors

The range of patients which nurses may be required to teach can be wide. The age, educational or occupational background and ethnicity of a patient population can be mixed and will require different approaches on the part of the educator.

Age

Many elderly individuals, in particular, are reported to have special educational needs (Johnston & Phil-

lipson, 1983), which relate to difficulties in concentrating or retaining material. Many elderly patients have perceptual problems or reduced manual dexterity. Furthermore, it may have been many years since they were required to undertake formal learning, resulting in diffidence and stress when learning new material or skills is required.

Language

Patients whose first language is not English may require special attention to ensure that material is readily comprehensible. This may include a slower pace of teaching and the inclusion of pictures or visual aids in educational material. Translation of information may help, although it is necessary to ascertain whether the individual reads as well as speaks their first language.

Literacy

Illiteracy is a difficulty which may confront the educator. It is estimated that as many as one individual in six may have literacy problems (Doak *et al.*, 1986). Education of such individuals requires special attention and skills, and identification of literacy problems may be complicated by the stigma associated with illiteracy and its consequent concealment.

Knowledge

Patients' prior knowledge, family history and experience can influence their learning needs and, perhaps more importantly, their expectations. Dealing with pre-conceptions about a patient's condition and its treatment can present a challenge to nurses engaged in patient education.

Disease

Many disease states are accompanied by physiological disturbances which can impact negatively upon learning. These include: impaired blood biochemistry and anaemia (e.g. in renal failure); hypoxia (e.g. in respiratory disease); and pain (which can accompany many chronic conditions). Allowance for the effects of these factors must be made in the preparation and execution of patient education programmes.

Mental state

Psychological disturbances are also commonplace in patients, particularly those who are newly diagnosed with a health problem (Morris, 1984; Turk, 1979). Anxiety and depression are common and can impair concentration and retention of material. Denial and grief can also impair an individual's ability to accept information. In addition, a patient's motivation to learn may be poor, particularly in cases where major changes in lifestyle are required.

Organisational factors

A number of organisational features can impinge upon the effectiveness of patient education. These include:

- Nursing skill mix
- Caseload mix
- Workload
- Educational resources
- Organisational support
- Peer support.

Nurse related factors

Research suggests that although most nurses recognise the importance of patient education, many avoid engaging in it or participate only reluctantly (Close, 1988). A number of factors appear to contribute to this.

Training
Training to undertake patient education does not form part of basic nurse education. Consequently, expectations that nurses should assess patients' learning needs and devise learning plans are unrealistic, since nurses are not normally equipped with the skills to undertake these tasks. Post-registration training in education is available in the shape of the relevant ENB course; however, this training does not specifically address the special educational needs of patients. This may also apply to the education component of such programmes as degrees and diplomas in nursing or community nursing.

Nursing philosophies
A further factor to be borne in mind concerns control over learning. The self-care philosophies underlying many chronic care programmes have the goal of promoting independence. It follows, therefore, that control over education would be in the hands of the patient, with the health care professionals acting primarily as resource persons and counsellors (Hasler, 1985; Walker, 1993). This may, however, conflict

with organisational goals and with the need to ensure patient safety by imparting a required minimum of information and skills. Certainly, many health care professionals, used themselves to didactic educational approaches and to being in control of patients' treatment programmes, may find this difficult.

However, work with long term patients and their carers remains an important aspect of the nurse's work in the community. Through patient education programmes the nurse has an opportunity to help improve patients' quality of life and maximise their health gain.

14.5 NURSE-RUN CLINICS

It has become increasingly commonplace in recent years for community nurses to run, more or less autonomously, clinics for screening and management of a number of chronic illnesses. In the United States, autonomous nurse-run community clinics are becoming a popular way of providing affordable health care and are a response to the country's problems with spiralling health care costs. In the United Kingdom, interest in nurse run clinics has been stimulated largely by the Government's 1990 contract for GPs (Department of Health, 1989).

This contract attempted to move away from the traditional capitation based fee for GPs and towards making payments on the basis of meeting a number of specific targets. Most of these targets relate to screening and preventative health care and marked a shift in policy on the part of Government. A noticeable result of the GP contract has been the surge in employment of nurses in general practices and the increased number of health promotion clinics, estimated by Hart (1993) to have been established subsequent to the contract by 93% of GPs. Much of the responsibility for health promotion and disease management clinics has been devolved to nurses.

The value of nurse-run clinics

The value of such clinics has been questioned (Stearn & Sullivan, 1993), not least because the structure of the clinics, the training of the staff and the input from other health care professionals can be so variable. The value of large scale screening programmes has been questioned. However, nurse-run clinics have some support and it is thought that they can be effective in promoting health and improving the management of chronic conditions such as asthma and diabetes (Gray, 1990; Charlton *et al.*, 1991). There is also evidence to suggest that, with appropriate training, nurses may actually perform such clinical procedures as blood pressure monitoring more accurately and reliably than doctors (Hart, 1993).

Not surprisingly, nurse-run clinics have gained widespread support from GPs, since it has enabled the delegation of many routine duties to the nurses (Charlton *et al.*, 1991). This has had some benefits for patients, since it has enabled more regular follow up and has encouraged the formulation of practice guidelines for nurses to follow, thus standardising practice (Fawcett, 1993; Gray, 1990). It has also found favour amongst nurses, since it has enabled some to find a role with flexible working hours and considerable autonomy (Scott, 1993).

However, enthusiasm for such clinics must be tempered with caution. Current evidence suggests that the training of nurses is at best patchy and that there is wide variability in the roles and responsibilities of nurses (Stearn & Sullivan, 1993). Many practice nurses have lacked job descriptions and have been required to do simply whatever the GP employing them has decided they should be doing, regardless of their skills or interests. It is important that nurses employ caution when taking on new roles and responsibilities, to ensure that the final outcome is a role which reflects their interests and skills and benefits patient's rather than being a result of doctors' desire to slough off boring and repetitive tasks, or worse, merely a way of providing services cheaply.

A number of case studies have been presented which detail the steps involved in establishing a nurse-run clinic. The series presented in the *British Journal of General Practice* by Charlton *et al.*, (1991) suggests that there are a number of important prerequisites:

- provision of appropriate training for nurses;
- allocation of suitable space;
- purchase of necessary equipment;
- development of protocols and guidelines for nurses;
- development of patient self-management strategies;

- development of patient education literature.

Training

There is a growing number of training courses, often run by private training agencies, aimed at nurses who are going to be running community based clinics. The quality of these is widely variable and they are often only short (e.g. three days or a week). Whilst this may be enough to give a general outline of the management of a particular health need or problem, it clearly cannot turn the nurse into a specialist in the area. The appropriateness of non-specialist community nurses, usually practice nurses, running disease-specific clinics, has therefore been questioned (Stearn & Sullivan, 1993). However, non-specialist nurses have also been employed in these roles with considerable success (Charlton *et al.*, 1991). It is apparent that as the community nurse's role evolves attention will need to be given to this aspect of nurse training.

Equipment

Provision of appropriate equipment may require financial outlay to ensure that patients can be supplied where necessary with monitoring devices such as sphygmomanometers and peak flow meters. It will also be necessary for nurses to become familiar with the recommended performance specifications for such devices. This will require reviewing the literature to find, if available, evidence of trials to support the reliability of a particular device (Beevers & Wilkins, 1987). Nurses should not merely rely upon company literature or the word of a sales representative, since it has been suggested that such information may not be sufficiently complete or research based (Hart, 1993).

Protocols

Development of protocols for the management of a particular condition is important to ensure that the care patients receive is efficient and standardised (Charlton *et al.*, 1991). Protocols also provide an important safeguard for nurses who are being required to act with relative autonomy, since there will be clear guidance as to the scope of their responsibilities and the appropriate point at which they should refer a patient on.

In practice, however, devising such protocols may

be easier said than done; for example, in the case of hypertension, there is on-going debate as to the thresholds for diagnosis and treatment of high blood pressure (Beevers & Wilkins, 1987; Hart, 1993). For some conditions, e.g. asthma and hypertension, guidelines for practice have been drawn up by expert panels: reference should be made to these where they are available. It seems likely that the use of clinical guidelines will become more commonplace in the future (Pearson, 1993). The practice is well established in the United States (Sharp, 1992), having been prompted into being by litigation consciousness, and despite some opposition from within the professions, clinical guidelines also have support at high levels in the United Kingdom.

Educational material

There is an increasing range of patient education material available for use by nurses, utilising diverse media, books and leaflets, videos, and computer software. Much of this literature is produced by drug companies and medical equipment manufacturers, and their imperative to promote their own products should always be borne in mind when reviewing such material. There is also some excellent patient information available from the voluntary patients' organisations and research bodies, such as the British Diabetic Association and the British Lung Foundation. The Health Education Authority is a further source of authoritative patient education literature. Special interest nurse groups also produce care outlines and educational literature. Such material is easily and usually quite cheaply acquired, and can be used by nurses responsible for running community clinics.

14.6 SUMMARY

Demographic changes in the population indicate that caring for chronically ill patients will form an increasing proportion of the work of community nurses. The care of such patients will require community nurses to adopt alternatives to the traditional nurse–patient relationship and to develop their skills in the area of patient education.

It is widely acknowledged that many patients do not follow their treatment regimens. Previously this was viewed in a negative light and often from a medical standpoint. Recent research has sought to explain so called non-compliance from the patient's perspective.

Self management of chronic health problems involves the patient being active in the treatment programme. Hence patients with long term problems will make judgements about the condition, its symptoms and control, and will weigh up the costs and benefits of a proposed regimen when deciding whether or not to follow professional advice.

Nurse-run clinics are one of the main places where community nurses come into contact with patients who have chronic illnesses. Nurse-run clinics have gained widespread support from GPs, since they have enabled GPs to delegate many routine duties. This in turn has led to benefits for patients since it has enabled more regular follow up and has to some extent standardised practice through the use of clinical guidelines.

14.7 REFERENCES AND FURTHER READING

Patient education

Ajzen, I. & Fishbein, M. (1980) *Understanding Attitudes and Predicting Social Behaviour* Prentice Hall, Englewood Cliffs.

Anderson, R. & Bury, M. (1988) *Living with Chronic Illness: the Experience of Patients and Their Families* Unwin Hyman, London.

Becker, M.H. & Maiman, L.A. (1975) Sociobehavioural determinants of compliance with health and medical care recommendations, *Medical Care*, **XIII**, 1, 10–24.

Bille, D.A. (1981) *Practical Approaches to Patient Teaching* Little, Brown and Co, Boston.

Boydell, T. (1985) *Experiential Learning* University of Manchester Press, Manchester.

Brearley, S. (1990) *Patient Participation: the Literature* (Royal College of Nursing Research Series). Scutari Press, Harrow, Middlesex.

Brookfield, S.D. (1986) *Understanding and Facilitating Adult Learning* Open University Press, Milton Keynes.

Charlton, I., Charlton, G., Broomfield, J. & Mullee, M.A. (1991) Audit of the effect of a nurse-run asthma clinic on workload and patient morbidity in general practice,

British Journal of General Practice, **41**, 227–31.

Close, A. (1988) Patient education: a literature review, *Journal of Advanced Nursing*, **13**, 203–13.

Doak, C.C., Doak, L.G. & Root, J.H. (1986) *Teaching Patients with Low Literacy Skills* J.B. Lippincott, Philadelphia.

Feely, M. & Pullar, T. (1989) Therapeutic compliance: myths and misunderstandings, *Geriatric Medicine*, **19**, 14–18.

Hasler, J.C. (1985) The very stuff of general practice, *Journal of the Royal College of General Practitioners*, **35**, 121–7.

Hermanova, H.M. (1985) Need for a database on consequences of disease, *International Rehabilitation Medicine*, **7**, 61–3.

Holland, S. (1986) Teaching patients and clients (part 1), *Nursing Times*, **82**, 49, 34–7.

Holland, S. (1987) Teaching patients and clients (part 2), *Nursing Times*, **83**, 3, 59–62.

Honey, P. & Mumford, A. (1982) *The Manual of Learning Styles* Ardingley House, Berkshire.

Johnston, S. & Phillipson, C. (1983) *Older Learners: The Challenge to Adult Education* Bedford Square Press, London.

Kidd, J.R. (1973) *How Adults Learn* Cambridge Books, New York.

Knowles, M.S. (1960) *The Handbook of Adult Education in the United States* Adult Education Association of the USA, Chicago.

Kolb, D.A. (1976) *Learning Styles Inventory: Technical Manual* McBer and Co., Boston.

Ley, P. (1982) Satisfaction, compliance and communication, *British Journal of Psychology*, **21**, 241–54.

Linn, M.W., Linn, B.S. & Stein, S.R. (1982) Satisfaction with ambulatory care and compliance in older adults, *Medical Care*, **XX**, 6, 606–14.

Locker, D. (1983) *Disability and Disadvantage: the Consequences of Chronic Illness* Tavistock, London.

Morris, J.E. (1984) Retreats from reality and pre-treatment education, *Journal of Nephrology Nursing*, **1**, 1, 54–7.

Redman, B.K. (1981) *Issues and Concepts in Patient Education* Appleton Century Crofts, New York.

Sackett, D. & Haynes, R.B. (1976) *Compliance with Therapeutic Regimens* Johns Hopkins University Press, Baltimore.

Stimson, G.V. (1974) Obeying doctor's orders: a view from the other side, *Social Science and Medicine*, **8**, 97–104.

Strauss, A.L. & Glaser, B.G. (1985) *Chronic Illness and the Quality of Life* Mosby, St Louis.

Tilley, J.D., Gregor, F.M. & Theissen, V. (1987) The nurse's role in patient education: incongruent perceptions amongst nurses and patients, *Journal of Advanced Nursing*, **12**, 291–301.

Turk, D.C. (1979) Factors influencing the adaptive process with chronic illness. In *Stress and Anxiety*, Volume 6 (Ed. by A. Sarason and C.D. Speilberger) Halsted Press, Washington DC.

Walker, R. (1993) Care and control of diabetes: finding the right balance, *Primary Health Care*, **3**, 10 16, 18, 20.

Wilson-Barnett, J. (1988) Patient teaching or patient counselling? *Journal of Advanced Nursing*, **13**, 215–22.

Zigmond, A.S. & Snaith, R.P.(1983) The hospital anxiety and depression scale, *Acta Psychiatrica Scandinavia*, **67**, 361–70.

Nurse-run clinics

Beevers, D.G. & Wilkins, M.R. (Ed) (1987) *The ABC of Hypertension* British Medical Association, London.

British Thoracic Society (1990a) Guidelines for the management of asthma in adults: I – chronic persistent asthma, *British Medical Journal*, **301**, 651–3.

British Thoracic Society (1990b) Guidelines for the management of asthma in adults: II – acute severe asthma, *British Medical Journal*, **301**, 797–800.

Charlton, I, Charlton, G., Broomfield, J. & Mullee, M.A. (1991) Audit of the effect of a nurse-run asthma clinic on workload and patient morbidity in general practice, *British Journal of General Practice*, **41**, 227–31.

Department of Health (1989) *Working for Patients. The Health Service: Caring for the 1990s* (Cmnd 555) HMSO, London.

Fawcett, H. (1993) Heartfelt advice, *Nursing Times*, **89**, 27, 36–8.

Gray, J. (1990) Promoting health in Tower Hamlets, *Senior Nurse*, **10**, 9, 26–8.

Hart, J.T. (1993) *Hypertension – Community Control of High Blood Pressure* (3rd ed) Radcliffe Medical Press, Oxford.

Pearson, M. (1993) Asthma guidelines: who is guiding whom and where to? *Thorax*, **48**, 197–8.

Petrie, J.C., O'Brien, E.T., Littler, W.A. & DeSwiet, M. (1986) British Hypertension Society: recommendations on blood pressure measurement, *British Medical Journal*, **293**, 611–15.

Scott, G. (1993) The path to good health, *Nursing Standard*, **7**, 44, 23.

Sharp, N. (1992) Six sets of clinical practice guidelines for 1992, *Nursing Management*, **23**, 11, 37–8.

Stearn, R. & Sullivan, F.M. (1993) Should practice nurses be involved in diabetic care? *British Journal of Nursing*, **2**, 19, 952–6.

Warner, J.O., Gotz, M. & Landau, L.I. (1992) Asthma: a follow-up statement from an International Paediatric Asthma Consensus Group, *Archives of Disease in Childhood*, **67**, 240–48.

Warner, J.O., Gotz, M. & Landau, L.I. (1989) Management of asthma: a consensus statement, *Archives of Disease in Childhood*, **64**, 1065–1079.

15

Management of HIV and AIDS

Caroline Carlisle

15.1 INTRODUCTION

In 1981, the first reports of a new set of symptoms, that was eventually to be called Acquired Immune Deficiency Syndrome (AIDS), appeared in North America. Cases of a rare form of pneumonia, pneumocystis carinii pneumonia (PCP) and an equally rare form of cancer, Kaposi's sarcoma (KS), were documented in young homosexual men. It was also noted that these men were immunodeficient, that is their immune system was damaged and inefficient. These diseases appeared to have been acquired and in 1983 the virus now known to cause AIDS was discovered. This virus has been given various names, but the internationally accepted term is now the human immunodeficiency virus (HIV). More recently another virus related to HIV has also been discovered in Africa. This new virus has been given the name HIV–2 and the original virus which is associated with the greatest number of cases of AIDS in the western world is now named HIV–1 (Ong, 1994).

Although originally identified amongst the homosexual population, it is now recognised that AIDS can affect all individuals regardless of gender, sexual orientation, age or race (Fan et al., 1994). In the early 1980s, however, the fact that HIV and AIDS was closely associated with groups who were already discriminated against within society, i.e. homosexual men and drug users, led to a societal response which was based on judgmental attitudes and further discrimination. As yet there is no cure for AIDS and although it has been noted that long term survival in HIV–1 infection is growing (Rutherford, 1994), the fear of HIV and AIDS has meant that both formal and informal carers have had to face the challenges of stigma and discrimination as well as meeting the physical and psychological needs of people affected by HIV.

Care in the home and community setting is particularly appropriate for people affected by HIV as it enables them to remain in familiar surroundings, so providing a strong basis for emotional support (Ungvarski & Nokes, 1992). Nearly all people with AIDS will require community nursing care at some point (Pratt, 1991).

The cause of AIDS and the spread of HIV

It is now known that AIDS is caused by HIV, but the spread of the virus still raises controversy over the means of transmission and the likelihood of transmission given exposure to the virus. The virus has been isolated from many body fluids, including saliva, tears and urine, although only blood, semen, vaginal and cervical secretions and breast milk have been directly implicated in the transmission of HIV. Numerous studies have been conducted in order to identify risk and prevalence of infection in a variety of circumstances. These studies include cohorts of injecting drug users (Ronald et al., 1993; Robertson et al., 1994), homosexual men (Evans, 1993), pregnant women (Nicoll, 1994), female sex workers (McKeganey et al., 1992) and patients attending an inner city accident and emergency department (Poznansky et al., 1994), to name but a few.

It is accepted that HIV infection is transmitted through sexual contact with infected persons and direct inoculation of contaminated blood products (Parris, 1992). There is also a risk of vertical transmission of the virus, that is perinatally from mother to neonate. There is also a risk, attributable to breast feeding, of transmission of the virus from an infected mother to her baby (Dunn *et al.*, 1992). Table 15.1 lists the means of transmission of HIV.

development of antibodies and when antibody positive. Although asymptomatic, the person is antibody positive after 45 days and a test to detect the antibodies can be carried out. This test is the routine one

Table 15.1 Means of transmission of HIV.

- **Sexual:** intimate sexual contact with an infected person via blood, cervical and vaginal fluid and semen.
- **Perinatally:** transplacental and during delivery.
- **Infected blood or blood products:** donor blood or blood products infected with HIV; injecting drug use through sharing needles and syringes contaminated with infected blood.
- **Organ transplantation; artificial insemination by donor semen.**

There are a number of difficulties in reporting the prevalence of HIV infection both nationally and globally. The fact that the incubation period is of variable duration and it can be as long as 8 to 10 years before any apparent signs and symptoms emerge (Fan *et al.*, 1994), means that the possibility exists that more people may be infected than are known about. Although there is potentially less difficulty in identifying people with AIDS, there can be a problem in the completeness of reporting of cases by medical practitioners (Evans *et al.*, 1991).

15.2 CLINICAL FEATURES OF HIV INFECTION AND AIDS

The majority of people who are exposed to HIV and become infected will not show signs of illness for a number of years due to the long incubation period of the virus. This is termed asymptomatic. They may feel well and only suspect that there is a possibility of being infected due to their risky behaviour or lifestyle. Some individuals experience mild 'flu-like symptoms or swollen glands shortly after initial infection but these are unspecific and cannot be taken as an indicator of HIV infection. During this asymptomatic period, antibodies to HIV are developed, usually by around 45 days after infection, but these do not prevent progression of the disease process. The individual is also potentially infectious to others prior to the

used to identify people who have been exposed to the virus.

HIV attacks and infects the very cells of the immune system that exist to fight off infection. The main cells which HIV affects are the T helper lymphocytes and macrophages. The cell receptor which HIV binds to is the CD4 surface protein which is present on T helper lymphocytes (Fan *et al.*, 1994). As HIV infection progresses, the number of helper cells decreases from a normal level of 800–1000 mm^3 to under 500 mm^3. Because of this, the body's normal response to infection is inhibited and the effect on the body can be wide ranging. Most of the physical symptoms which can develop, sometimes not until ten years or longer after the initial infection, are the indirect result of damage to the immune system by HIV. Initial symptoms can include enlarged lymph glands (persistent generalised lymphadenopathy (PGL)), fevers and night sweats. Signs and symptoms of opportunistic infections can develop. Opportunistic infections are so called because they are infections with pathogens which normally our immune systems can fight off with no difficulty. They only become a problem when the immune system is not working properly.

In addition, HIV can have direct effects upon the body, for example by attacking the cells in the brain and this can lead to HIV encephalopathy. Brain function can then be impaired to various degrees and this can range from lack of concentration to personality changes and disorders of motor function. Eventual effects on the brain can be major intellectual incapacity and motor disability.

Cancers can also develop, the most common of which is either Kaposi's sarcoma (KS) or non-Hodgkin's malignant lymphoma. KS presents as dark, purplish or brown lesions which can be located on the arms, legs or in the mouth. KS lesions can also involve visceral organs such as the lungs, liver and gastro-intestinal tract.

The eventual diagnosis of AIDS in a person who is HIV positive is not made by any one single test. A variety of signs and symptoms are explored before a person is given an AIDS diagnosis. The disorders which can lead to this diagnosis are often termed AIDS defining disorders and they by no means have the same prognosis or outlook for the HIV positive person. It has been suggested that the term AIDS is obsolete and the use of a broader diagnostic term such as HIV disease is more appropriate (Volberding,

1989). The ways in which an AIDS diagnosis has been reached have also evolved over the lifetime of our knowledge of HIV and the Centre for Disease Control in Atlanta provides an up to date classification scheme. Table 15.2 outlines the possible progression of symptoms in HIV disease.

15.3 GUIDANCE FOR PRACTICE – PRIMARY PREVENTION

Primary prevention is the aspect of care which deals with the achievement of the full health potential of the individual. This can involve identification of people

Table 15.2 Possible progression of symptoms in HIV disease.

Exposure to virus and initial infection

These are relatively mild disease symptoms which appear prior to seroconversion and usually last only a few days and then disappear.
Flu like illness, joint and muscle pains, sore throat, skin rash, swollen lymph glands (generalised lymphadenopathy).
Brain inflammation, headache and fever, difficulty in concentrating, memory problems.

Asymptomatic period

Although asymptomatic, the patient is infectious throughout this period. This stage can last up to 12 years.

Initial symptoms

Patients can experience a mixture of any of these symptoms.
Wasting syndrome (sudden and unexplained loss of more than 10% of total body weight), night sweats and fevers.
Persistant generalised lymphadenopathy (PGL).
Neurological disease, can present as dementia, myelopathy, weakness, paralysis, altered sensation in limbs.

Early immune failure

Some of the more opportunistic infections can occur during this phase.
Oral candidiasis (thrush), seborrhoeic dermatitis, hairy leucoplakia (unique to HIV infection), herpes zoster (shingles), tinea pedis (athletes foot), condyloma acuminata (genital warts).

AIDS

This presents as some of the major opportunistic infections and/or secondary cancers.
Pneumocystis carinii pneumonia (the major cause of death in people with AIDS), protozoan infections, bacterial infections, fungal infections, viral infections such as cytomegalovirus which can lead to blindness, pneumonia and gastroenteritis.
Cancers such as Kaposi's sarcoma (KS) and lymphomas.

with risk behaviours associated with HIV transmission and health education focused on risk reduction. Community nurses can be involved at this level in either the clinic or home setting. The majority of health education undertaken in the community will be on a one-to-one basis and the individualised nature of this makes it amongst the most valuable and reliable (While, 1983).

Assessment of health needs: HIV specific

The taking of an HIV-specific health history should be done in an atmosphere of confidentiality, trust and with a non–judgmental approach. The history will, of necessity, address what can be intimate and normally private aspects of a person's life and an accurate assessment will help direct the most appropriate information and advice giving. Accuracy can only be achieved if the patient feels trust and any limits to confidentiality have been made explicit.

When taking a health history the nurse should avoid making any assumptions about the patient's risk potential for HIV. The focus should be on any potentially risky behaviour rather than on 'at risk' groups which are generally already stigmatised in society.

The history should include the following:

Sexual behaviour
This is not simply the identification of sexual preference but an assessment of the specific sexual behaviour that can potentially increase the risk of HIV transmission between two people. Condom use should be carefully assessed and questions should address the type of condom used, whether an appropriate water-based lubricant is used and whether the patient knows how to use a condom properly.

Patients' perspectives on their own risk behaviour
It is essential to assess what patients see as the risks within their own lifestyle or behaviour. In this way the 'worried well' can be identified and reassurances given about the levels of risk to which they feel they have been exposed.

Patients' perspectives on their own clinical symptoms
Many of the early signs and symptoms of HIV related illness are non-specific and many can present without HIV infection, e.g. thrush, herpes simplex. The nurse should, however, listen to the patient's concerns and,

taking the rest of the history into consideration, reach realistic conclusions with regard to the potential for clinical symptoms to be HIV related.

Drug use
This should include, where appropriate, an assessment of the ways in which drugs are used and the procedures which patients are following with regard to safety, e.g. whether sharing of 'works' (needles, syringes, etc.) takes place.

Occupational history
There may be concerns regarding accidental exposure to blood, other body fluids and needles. It is also essential to check on any follow-up care and investigation which has taken place since any accidental exposure, e.g. after accidental inoculation due to needle stick injury.

Medical history and examination
It is important to distinguish between those patients who present as 'worried well' and those who have symptoms of physical illness. The former are unlikely to require the nurse to take anything other than a brief medical history in order to confirm that their needs are primarily for information, advice and reassurance. Where necessary, however, a full medical history should be obtained and this should include specific questions related to:

- current/past medication, particularly the use of any drugs which suppress the immune system;
- current/past disease and illness, including sexually transmitted diseases, haemophilia, tuberculosis;
- transfusion or organ transplant;
- surgical treatments.

Medical examination should encompass a general review of all the systems. Given that HIV can affect virtually every body system, it is essential that this physical examination is thorough and comprehensive. If a nurse has not been specifically educated in physical examination, then referral must be made to the appropriate medical practitioner.

Implementing care

The needs of the patient at this time will be for accurate information, appropriate advice giving and for non-directive support relating to issues around lifestyle and behaviour. It may be more appropriate for the patient to be referred to expert sources of support and guidance. Every nurse should be aware of his or her own limitations when it comes to caring for people who are worried or affected by HIV/AIDS. Where necessary, referral to specialist support clinics and practitioners should be offered.

Information giving

The information offered should be related to the patient's particular needs and this can cover the following:

- Transmission of HIV and those body fluids which are known to transmit the virus
- Guidelines for safer sexual practices. The provision of information on risky and less risky sexual practices can be seen at one level to be rather simplistic. All explanations of safer sexual behaviour must take into account attitudes, values and patients' own perspectives on their sexuality and the extent of their power within current sexual relationships. For example, many women who identify as lesbians see condoms as irrelevant to their sexual practices (Squire, 1993). It may be more appropriate and helpful for the patient to be referred to one of the specialist HIV/AIDS agencies or telephone helplines (see Section 15.8)

where information and advice can be given which is focused on the specific needs of that patient. Table 15.3 provides general guidelines on risk in relation to sexual practices.

- HIV testing facilities. The majority of nurses in the community have not been specifically prepared to offer HIV pre-test counselling and patients who are considering testing should, therefore, be referred to an appropriate clinic or agency. Nurses should, however, be able to provide local information on the following:
  - addresses, telephone numbers and clinic times, including a selection of hospital and community based clinics;
  - clinics which offer same day test and results;
  - single sex clinics;
  - basic information on ways in which confidentiality is maintained at clinics;
  - whether a testing guide is available. (Some agencies have produced an evaluation of the locally available clinics and their facilities; information on this would be obtainable from local HIV/AIDS agencies.)

Non-directive support

The sensitive and private nature of the worries and concerns which HIV raises, calls for the implementation of both basic and advanced communication

Table 15.3 Guidelines on levels of risk related to different sexual practices. (The risk differs in relation to sexual practices depending on the frequency of the practice, the HIV status of a sexual partner, and other co-factors such as state of health and drug use.)

High risk activities

Unprotected anal or vaginal sexual intercourse (e.g. without a condom).
Sharing sex toys without appropriate cleaning.
Traumatic sexual activity, e.g. fisting (manual-anal insertion), as this can cause damage to mucosa prior to sexual intercourse.
Oral sex on a man who ejaculates into your mouth.

Lower risk activities

Protected anal or vaginal sexual intercourse (e.g. using a condom).
Oral sex using condom or dental dam (4 inch square latex sheet).

Least risky activities

Non-insertive sexual practices, e.g. mutual masturbation.
Dry kissing (closed mouth), hugging, caressing, non-genital licking.

skills on the part of the nurse. The following are the core skills which should be part of all communication with those worried or affected by HIV:

- Confidentiality: the patient should be made aware of any limits to confidentiality and the ways in which records, if any, are held and who has access to these. All information related to patients should be led by a 'need to know' policy and the patient should, wherever possible, be in control of this.
- Non-judgmental approach: the stigma associated with HIV/AIDS poses many problems for patients. Nurses should be aware of their own prejudices and refer patients to other avenues of support and help if they feel their own attitudes may restrict the psychological support they can provide for any patient. There is, however, a duty to care and nurses should at all times strive to offer care in an atmosphere of respect.
- Listening skills: active listening involves conveying to patients that your attention is focused on them and on the issues as seen from their perspective. Conveying active listening can be done through the use of appropriate eye contact and touch, reflecting and paraphrasing skills, and body posture. Probably the most effective means whereby care at this level is conveyed is in the giving of time; time which is specifically for listening and not for the carrying out of practical tasks.

15.4 GUIDANCE FOR PRACTICE – SECONDARY PREVENTION

Secondary prevention is implemented as soon as HIV infection is diagnosed. The goal at this stage is one of maintaining or improving the patient's psychological and physical wellbeing, and should include providing information on ways to avoid the spread of the virus. It has to be remembered that the patient may well be asymptomatic and be grappling with decisions related to the possible commencement of anti-viral drug therapy, e.g. zidovudine (AZT). Community staff may have limited contact with patients at this stage unless working as part of a specialist community

HIV/AIDS team. The most likely contact may well be immediately after the diagnosis of the positive status of the patient, i.e. after receiving HIV test results. It may be that professional contact with the partner, friends or family of the positive person can lead to the need for care to be directed towards the support of the significant other.

Psychological support

A positive test result can be an overwhelming experience for many people and the resultant shock, denial, fear, and loss can cause severe psychological trauma (Ungvarski, 1992). There may also be feelings of guilt at the possibility of having infected others with the virus. Worries around stigmatisation may be present and although the patient may not have experienced discrimination from others, the perception that it can happen is extremely stressful. The experience of a positive result is an awareness of a sudden and radical change in life; a life that is now lived in uncertainty by infected patients (Pierret, 1992) and their families (Brown & Powell-Cope, 1991).

A number of appropriate referral points may be suggested to a patient at this stage. It is unlikely that a community nurse who does not specialise in HIV/AIDS will be able to meet the full range of psychological needs of the patient. Referrals can be made to other members of the health care team, including community psychiatric nurses. Amongst the most useful referrals are likely to be to the following:

- Specialist HIV/AIDS counsellors: this service is often provided by local sexually transmitted diseases clinics, non-statutory/voluntary HIV/AIDS agencies, or specialist health care teams.
- Self help groups: agencies such as Body Positive provides a support service given by HIV positive people for positive people (see Section 15.8, Appendix: Specialist Referral Agencies).
- Buddies: a buddy is a volunteer who is normally trained and works for voluntary HIV/AIDS agencies (see Section 15.8 Appendix: Specialist Referral Agencies), and is able to provide a befriending service to positive people. The buddy is 'matched' to a positive person and can provide support and friendship to the person and significant others in his or her life.

Tertiary prevention is concerned with the nursing care which is required for a person with advancing HIV related disease, including the clinical signs and symptoms associated with AIDS. The following guidelines highlight some of the main areas with which community nurses may have to deal. Given the wide ranging effect of HIV on the body, patients will present with a variety of clinical signs and symptoms.

Assessment and planning

The assessment should be systematic and take a holistic approach including the physical, psychological, social and spiritual aspects. The needs of other carers such as family, friends or significant others will need to be addressed.

Assessment involves liaison with other members of the health care team, such as the GP, and formal and informal carers. If the patient is to be discharged from hospital it is important that both professionals and carers are involved in the discharge planning process in order to maintain consistency in the services offered to the patient. The hospital and/or specialists involved in the care of the patient are an essential source of support and guidance not only for the patient but also for community nursing staff.

The needs of the patient should be addressed from the patient's perspective. The care plan should be drawn up with the full involvement of the patient and any informal carers who are involved.

Community nurses are in an important position with regard to co-ordination of services and appropriate referral to specialist support.

Implementation of care

Much of the care which the community nurse will provide is similar to that needed by any seriously ill patient being cared for at home. This section will present guidelines on those aspects of care which are not normally a major part of the community nurse's role. The implementation of care in the community also involves providing information, advice and health teaching to those informal carers who will be giving care between visits. Many of their concerns will be around practical care issues and safety with regard to the transmission of the virus.

Infection control

'Universal precautions' is the term used to signify those precautions which apply to blood and to other body fluids containing visible blood. It also applies to semen and vaginal secretions, although these fluids have not been implicated in occupational transmission from patient to nurse. Other body fluids included are cerebro-spinal fluid, synovial fluid, pleural fluid, peritoneal fluid, pericardial fluid and amniotic fluid. The basis of universal precautions is one where the blood and certain body fluids of *all patients*, regardless of what is known or not known about their viral status (e.g. HIV, hepatitis B, hepatitis C, etc.), are considered potentially infectious. The guidelines which follow are mainly based on the Center for Disease Control Recommendations (1987):

- Ensure all cuts and or abrasions are covered with a water-proof dressing whilst on duty.

- Effective hand-washing technique should be practised before and after all patient contact. Jewellery which interferes with effective hand-washing should not be worn.

- Use protective barriers such as gloves, masks and gowns appropriately.

   Disposable latex gloves and disposable aprons should be worn when dealing with bedpans and urinals. Gloves should also be worn for venepuncture, for touching mucous membranes or non-intact skin of patients, and for handling items or surfaces which are soiled with blood or body fluids.

   Disposable aprons should be worn only during procedures that are likely to generate splashes of blood or other body fluids.

   Masks or protective eyewear should be worn only during procedures that may generate droplets of blood or body fluids such as suctioning or if the patient is coughing excessively.

- If hands are contaminated with body fluids, wash immediately with a chlorhexidine gluconate solution such as Hibiscrub.

■ Take precautions to prevent injuries caused by needles, and other sharps. Used needles are never re-sheathed, bent or broken and are disposed of promptly in rigid, puncture resistant, leak proof sharps containers which must not be more than three quarters filled before being sealed and taken for incineration.

　　Use of a closed system such as the monovette system for venepuncture is a safe and effective way to help avoid accidental inoculation.

■ Spillages of blood and other body fluids should be dealt with by an appropriate disinfection procedure, e.g. granules of NaDCC (sodium dichloroisocyanurate). 'Presept' granules or a solution of household bleach (1:10 solution), should be used to cover the spillage for 10 minutes and then carefully wiped up with disposable paper towels whilst wearing gloves.

　　Used dressings contaminated with blood or body fluids should be disposed of in heavy duty yellow plastic bags with effective ties for closure. Arrangements should be made for discrete collection and incineration according to local arrangements for the disposal of infected waste.

　　Linen which has been contaminated by blood and body fluids can be washed using the household washing machine, on the hot cycle wash (71°C) using normal detergent. If laundry services are required, the linen should be placed in a water soluble bag (e.g. algenate bag) before being placed in a secondary red nylon bag. Arrangements should be made for discrete collection according to local arrangements, generally by the environmental health department.

Appropriate guidance with regard to universal precautions must be given to informal carers at home. It is also important to emphasise that sharing bathrooms and kitchens poses no risk. No special disinfectants are required for baths, toilets or sinks other than those normally used. No separate cutlery and crockery is normally required.

Intravenous drug therapy (IVT)

The option of IVT for patients at home has greatly increased the quality of life for people with AIDS. The need to attend clinics or to be admitted to acute care units is reduced and the patient can remain in the home environment for longer periods of time. Most people with AIDS will require IVT at some time in order to administer chemotherapy, antibiotics or blood and nutritional therapy.

There is also a growing use of central venous catheters (e.g. Hickman lines or Portacaths) for the administration of primary and secondary prophylaxis.

It is essential that all community nurses who may be required to administer and supervise IVT in the home receive adequate training, particularly relating to asepsis in a non-clinical environment and patient self-administration (English National Board, 1994).

It is recommended that there should be local updating facilities for IVT administration that can be arranged at short notice once a potential discharge from hospital is notified (Oliver, 1992).

Neurological effects of HIV

Neurological problems related to HIV can be due to a variety of causes such as opportunistic infection (e.g. cytomegalovirus), cerebral haemorrhage or Kaposi's sarcoma lesions. Chronic HIV related encephalopathy is one of the major causes of neurological dysfunction. This encephalopathy is often referred to as AIDS dementia. Symptoms include: progressive cognitive dysfunction with inability to concentrate; decreased memory; motor deficits such as leg weakness or ataxia; and behaviourial changes such as social withdrawal or aggression. The end stage usually results in the person being doubly incontinent and being unable to walk.

Community nurses are well placed to recognise the initial signs of AIDS dementia such as memory and concentration problems or taking longer to complete activities of living. Note should be taken when informal carers comment on any signs which may suggest neurological problems.

The goals of care should be to promote independence, minimise disorientation and provide for safety. Implementation of care should involve the following:

Safety
The patient may have poor balance and be uncoordinated, which can result in falls or dropping things. The home environment will need to be accurately assessed for safety and any modifications planned with the collaboration of the patient and informal carers.

Patients may display aggressive behaviour both toward community staff and informal carers. Decisions with regard to the appropriate environment for care in these instances should be carried out after full assessment and taking into account the needs and wants of both the patient and informal carer.

Orientation
Where appropriate, health education of informal carers about ways to help orientate the patient in place and time can be given. Using clocks, watches and calendars, reading the newspaper to the patient, and listening to the radio are all helpful ways to orientate regularly.

Communication
Verbal and non-verbal techniques for communicating with people who are confused, disorientated or

deal of time in order that the required level of support is provided so that they can continue to care. Respite care should be offered where appropriate.

Physical care
This will depend on the extent of neurological impairment, but can include assistance with all activities of living.

Other clinical symptoms

The patient can present with clinical symptoms related to a variety of opportunistic infections, complications of drug therapy, or malignancies. Table 15.4 outlines some of the common signs and symptoms with which a community nurse may have to deal.

Table 15.4 HIV related disease: common clinical symptoms and causes.

Symptom	Possible causes
Weight loss	Opportunistic infection, anorexia and vomiting due to side effects of medication, mouth infection.
Lethargy and fatigue	Opportunistic infections or malignancies, anaemia, malnutrition, diarrhoea.
Dry skin and skin lesions	Shingles, herpes simplex, dermatitis, candida albicans infection, immobility, malnutrition.
Dry and painful mouth	Candida albicans, herpes simplex, malnutrition.
Diarrhoea	Gastro-intestinal infection, KS lesions in gastro-intestinal tract.
Breathlessness and cough	Pneumocystis carinii pneumonia, KS lesions in respiratory tract.
Oedema	Lymphatic occlusion by HIV or opportunistic viral infection.
Impaired vision	Chorioretinitis due to opportunistic infection.
Pain	Malignancies, myopathy, opportunistic infection.

demented should be implemented where appropriate and informal carers assisted with these techniques also.

It is important to continue to communicate and to involve the patient in decision making with regard to care whenever possible.

Basic communication skills should be employed and this should include active listening, the provision of time to talk, and clarity with regard to information and/or instructions for such things as medication.

Informal carers in the home will also need a great

15.6 SUMMARY

Improved management of HIV related disease means that patients spend over 80% of their time in the community setting (Layzell & McCarthy, 1993). It is likely that community nurses will come into contact at some point with people affected or infected by HIV. The nature of HIV and AIDS means that care will be required at primary, secondary and tertiary prevention stages and that holistic care planning must involve not only the people infected but those who care for them, i.e. family, partners, friends.

Community staff may have to deal at a primary prevention stage with people who are 'worried well' or who wish to have information on prevention of spread of the virus. The skills required here will primarily be those of patient education, communication and keeping up-to-date with knowledge about the virus.

When someone is diagnosed as HIV positive it is important that the most appropriate information is given regarding care and referrals. A multidisciplinary approach is essential and this should involve non-statutory and voluntary agencies who specialise in HIV/AIDS related support.

Advancing HIV related disease will call on the full range of the community nurse's skills in order to meet the physical and psychological needs of the patient and family or significant others. All care planning must involve the collaboration of the patient and any informal carers.

Community nurses are in an ideal position to co-ordinate and meet the needs of people affected or infected by HIV. Nurses caring in this area must be adequately prepared.

15.7 REFERENCES AND FURTHER READING

Brown, M.A. & Powell-Cope, G.M. (1991) AIDS family caregiving: transitions through uncertainty, *Nursing Research*, **40**, 6, 338–45.

Center for Disease Control (1987) Recommendations for preventing HIV transmission in health care settings, *Morbidity and Mortality Weekly Report*, **36** (Supp.), 1S–18S.

Dunn, D.T., Newell, M.L., Ades, A.E. & Peckham, C.S. (1992) Risk of human immunodeficiency virus type 1 transmission through breastfeeding. *The Lancet*, **340**, 585–8.

English National Board for Nursing, Midwifery and Health Visiting (1994) *The HIV/AIDS Education and Training Project, Final Report of the Working Group on 'Developing the Role of the District Nurse in the Administration of Intravenous Therapy in the Home'*. English National Board, London.

Evans, B.G., Gill, O.N. & Emslie, J.A.N. (1991) Com-

pleteness of reporting of AIDS cases, *British Medical Journal*, **302**, 1351–2.

Evans, B.G., Catchpole, M.A., Heptonstall, J., Mortimer, J.Y., McCarrigle, C.A., Nicoll, A.G., Waight, P., Gill, O.N., Swan, A.V. (1993) Sexually transmitted diseases and HIV–1 infection among homosexual men in England and Wales, *British Medical Journal*, **306**, 426–8.

Fan, H., Conner, R.F. & Villarreal, L.P. (1994) *The Biology of AIDS* (3rd ed.), Jones and Bartlett Publishers, London.

Layzell, S. & McCarthy, M. (1993) Specialist or generic community nursing care for HIV/AIDS patients? *Journal of Advanced Nursing*, **18**, 531–7.

McKeganey, N., Barnard, M., Leyland, A., Coote, I. & Follet, E. (1992) Female streetworking prostitution and HIV infection in Glasgow, *British Medical Journal*, **305**, 801–804.

Nicoll, A., McGarrigle, C., Heptonstall, J., Parry, J., Mahoney, A., Nicholas, S., Hutchinson, E. & Gill, O.N. (1994) Prevalence of HIV infection in pregnant women in London and elsewhere in England, *British Medical Journal*, **309**, 376–7.

Oliver, G. (1992) Intravenous line care at home, *Primary Health Care*, **1**, 5, 12–16.

Ong, E. (1994) Infection with the human immunodeficiency virus: an overview, *Care of the Critically Ill*, **9**, 1, 7–10.

Parris, N.B. (1992) Infection control. In *HIV/AIDS: A Guide to Nursing Care* (Ed. by J.H. Flaskerud and P.J. Ungvarski) (2nd ed.), W.B. Saunders, Philadelphia.

Pierret, J. (1992) Coping with AIDS in everyday life. In *AIDS: a Problem for Sociological Research* (Ed. by M. Pollak, G. Paicheter & J. Pierret) Sage Publications, London

Poznansky, M.C., Torkington, J., Turner, G., Bankes, M.J.K., Parry, J.V., Connell, J.A., Touquet, R. Weber, J. (1994) Prevalence of HIV infection in patients attending an inner city accident and emergency department, *British Medical Journal*, **308**, 636.

Pratt, R. (1991) *AIDS: a Strategy for Nursing Care*. Edward Arnold, London.

Robertson, J.R., Ronald, P.J.M., Raab, G.M., Ross, A.J. & Parpia, T. (1994) Deaths, HIV infection, abstinence, and other outcomes in a cohort of injecting drug users followed up for 10 years, *British Medical Journal*, **309**, 369–72.

Ronald, P.J.M., Robertson, J.R., Wyld, R. & Weightman, R. (1993) Heterosexual transmission of HIV in injecting drug users, *British Medical Journal*, **307**, 1184–5.

Rutherford, G.W. (1994) Long term survival in HIV–1 infection, *British Medical Journal*, **309**, 283–94.

Squire, C. (1993) *Women and AIDS: Psychological Perspectives*. Sage Publications, London.

Ungvarski, P.J. & Nokes, K.M. (1992) Community-based and long-term care. In *HIV/AIDS: a Guide to Nursing*

Care (Ed. by J.H. Flaskerud & P.J. Ungvarski) (2nd edn). W.B. Saunders Company, Philadelphia.

Ungvarski, P.J. (1992) Nursing management of the adult client. In *HIV/AIDS: a Guide to Nursing Care* (Ed. by J.H. Flaskerud & P.J. Ungvarski (2nd ed.). W.B. Saunders & Company, Philadelphia.

Volberding, P.A. (1989) HIV infection as a disease: the medical indications for early diagnosis, *The Journal of Acquired Immune Deficiency Syndrome*, **2**, 5, 421–6.

While, A.E. (1983) Teaching those in need in the community. In *Patient Teaching: Recent Advances in Nursing 6* (Ed. by J. Wilson-Barnett) Churchill Livingstone, Edinburgh.

15.8 APPENDIX: SPECIALIST REFERRAL AGENCIES

There is a wide variety of agencies which provide services for all people affected by HIV/AIDS. Only a few are included in this appendix. Should you be in any doubt whether an agency exists for the needs of your patient/client a call to any local or national AIDS helpline should provide you with accurate up-to-date information on potential referral agencies.

By far the most comprehensive and accurate source of information on all aspects of HIV/AIDS is the *National AIDS Manual* (NAM), which is published by NAM Publications Ltd, Unit 52, Eurolink Centre, 49 Effra Road, London SW2 1BZ. Telephone: (0171) 737-1846. A yearly subscription includes three updates during the year. It is published in three volumes which comprise: *Topics, Directory of Agencies*, and *Treatments and Trials*.

Support groups

The following agencies provide a range of services for people affected by HIV and AIDS. The contact numbers and the services provided are correct at the time of publication, but it would be advisable to check prior to passing the telephone number on to a patient/client.

Body Positive, 51b Philbeach Gardens, Earls Court, London SW5 9EB. The network telephone number is 01582-484887 and they would be able to provide any local regional telephone number of groups outside of London. This is a self-help group for people affected by HIV/AIDS and offers a wide range of services and self-help. The telephone helplines are answered by men and women who are themselves HIV positive.

Positively Women, 5 Sebastian Street, London EC1V

OHE. Office: (0171) 490-5501; client services: (0171) 490-5515. 10 am–5 pm. Local regional numbers can be obtained by calling either of these lines.
This agency provides a range of free and confidential counselling and support services to women with AIDS, HIV, or any of the associated conditions.

Terrence Higgins Trust, 52–54 Grays Inn Road, London WC1X 8JU. Telephone (0171) 831-0330. 9.30 am–6 pm. Helpline: (0171) 242-1010. 12 noon–10pm.
This aims to provide welfare, legal and counselling help and support, including a Buddies service and Family Support Network. It also provides health education about HIV/AIDS.

MacFarlane Trust, PO Box 627, London SW1H OQG. Helpline: (0171) 233-0342. Mon–Fri, 9 am–5 pm.
This Trust aims to help people (and their dependants) with haemophilia who were infected with HIV as a result of their treatment for haemophilia.

Centres and hospices

Bethany, St Mary's Road Bodmin, Cornwall PL31 1NF. Telephone 01208-79035.
This is a house of rest and respite for people with HIV and AIDS, their families, carers and friends. If offers short term care for up to a maximum of six weeks and has family, double, twin and single bedrooms.

London Lighthouse, 111–117 Lancaster Road, London Wll lQT. Telephone (0171) 792-1200.
The London Lighthouse is a residential and support centre for people affected by AIDS and provides a comprehensive range of services, including a drop-in centre, legal and welfare advice, counselling and support services, day care and home support. The residential unit provides clinical care in a non-institutionalised environment.

Mildmay Mission Hospital, Hackney Road, London E2 7NA. Telephone: (0171) 739-2331.
This is an independent Christian charitable hospital specialising in palliative care services for all people affected by AIDS. It also has a home care team, a family unit and a day care unit.

Table of Statutes

Health and Safety at Work Act 1974
Medicines Act 1968
Misuse of Drugs Act 1971
National Health Service and Community Care Act 1990
Poisons Act 1972

Statutory Instruments

SI 1985 No. 2066 Misuse of Drugs Regulations 1985
SI 1973 No. 798 Misuse of Drugs Act (Safe Storage Regulations) 1973

Useful Addresses

Action for Dysphasic Adults,
1, Royal Street,
London SE1 7LN.
Telephone: 0171 261 9572.

Age Concern,
Astral House,
1268, London Road,
London SW16 4ER.
Telephone: 0181 679 8000.

AIDS Support Groups and Agencies,
See Appendix,
Chapter 15.

Alzheimers Disease Society,
10, Green Coat Place,
London SW1P 1PH.
Telephone: 0171 306 0606.

Arthritis Care,
18, Stevenson Way,
London NW1 2HD.
Telephone: 0171 916 1500.

Association for Continence Advice,
The Basement,
2, Doughty Street,
London WC1N 2PN.
Telephone: 0171 404 6821.

British Association for Counselling,
1, Regent Place,
Rugby CV21 2PJ.
Telephone: 01788 578328.

British College of Acupuncture,
8, Hunter Street,
London WC1N 1BN.
Telephone: 0171 833 8164.

British Colostomy Association,
38–39, Eccleston Square,
London SW1V 1PB.
Telephone: 0171 828 5175.

British Diabetic Association,
10, Queen Anne Street,
London W1M 0BD.
Telephone: 0171 323 1531.

British Heart Foundation,
14, Fitzhardinge Street,
London W1H 4DH.
Telephone: 0171 935 0185.

British Hypertension Society,
185, Uxbridge Road,
Hampton,
Middlesex TW12 1BN.
Telephone: 0181 783 0810.

British Hypnotherapy Association,
67, Upper Berkley Street,
London W1H 7DH.
Telephone: 0171 723 4443.

British Thoracic Society,
1, St Andrew's Place,
Regents Park,
London NW1 4LB.
Telephone: 0171 486 7766.

Cancer Relief Macmillan Fund,
15–19, Britten Street,
London SW3 3TZ.
Telephone: 0171 351 7811.

Cancer Research Campaign,
6–10, Cambridge Terrace,
London NW1 4JL.
Telephone: 0171 224 1333.

Carers' National Association,
20–25, Glasshouse Yard,
London EC1A 4JS.
Telephone: 0171 490 8818.

Chartered Society of Physiotherapists,
14, Bedford Row,
London WC1R 4ED.
Telephone: 0171 606 2435.

Consumers Association,
2, Marylebone Road,
London NW1 4DF.
Telephone: 0171 486 5544.

Continence Foundation,
The Basement,
2, Doughty Street,
London WC1N 2PN.
Telephone: 0171 404 6875.

Coronary Prevention Group,
Plantation House,
31–35, Fenchurch Street,
London EC3M 3NN.
Telephone: 0171 626 4844.

CRUSE Bereavement Care,
Cruse House,
126, Sheen Road,
Richmond TW9 1UR.
Telephone: 0181 940 4818.

Disabled Living Foundation,
286, Camden Road,
London N7 0BJ.
Telephone: 0171 289 6111.

Headway – National Head Injuries Association
200, Mansfield Road,
Nottingham NG1 3HX.
Telephone: 01602 622382.

Health & Safety Executive,
1–3, Chepstow Place,
Westbourne Grove,
London W1 4TF.
Telephone: 0171 229 3456.

Health Education Authority,
78, New Oxford Street,
London WC1A 1AH
Telephone: 0171 383 3833.

HIV Support Groups and Agencies,
See Appendix,
Chapter 15.

Homeopathic Trust,
2, Powis Place,
London WC1.
Telephone: 0171 837 9469.

Incontact
National Action on Incontinence
Confidential Helpline.
Telephone: 0191 213 0050.

Institute for Complementary Medicine,
21, Portland Place,
London W1N 3AF.
Telephone: 0171 237 5165.

International Multiple Sclerosis Society,
10, Haddon Street,
London W1R 7LJ.
Telephone: 0171 734 9120.

Leg Ulcer Forum,
Parsons Green Centre,
5–7, Parsons Green,
London SW6 4UT.
Telephone: 0181 846 6767.

Marie Curie Cancer Care,
28, Belgrave Square,
London SW1X 8QG.
Telephone: 0171 235 3325.

National Back Pain Association,
16, Elm Tree Road,
Teddington,
Middlesex TW11 8ST.
Telephone: 0181 977 5474.

National Pharmaceutical Association,
38–42, St Peter's Street,
St Albans,
Herts AL1 3NP.
Telephone: 01727 832161.

Royal College of Nursing,
20, Cavendish Square,
London W1M 0AB.
Telephone: 0171 872 0840.

Royal National Institute for the Blind,
224, Great Portland Street,
London W1N 6AA.
Telephone: 0171 388 1266.

Royal National Institute for the Deaf,
105, Gower Street,
London WC1E 6AH.
Telephone: 0171 387 8033.

Stroke Association,
CHSA House,
Whitecross Street,
London EC1Y 8JJ.
Telephone: 0171 490 7999.

UKCC,
23, Portland Place,
London W1N 3AF.
Telephone: 0171 637 7181.

Index

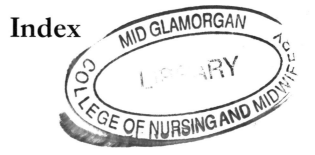

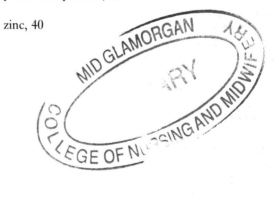